....
Street Foods

World Review of Nutrition and Dietetics

Vol. 86

KARGER   Basel · Freiburg · Paris · London · New York ·
New Delhi · Bangkok · Singapore · Tokyo · Sydney

Street Foods

Volume Editors

A.P. Simopoulos
The Center for Genetics, Nutrition and Health,
Washington, D.C.
R.V. Bhat
National Institute of Nutrition,
Indian Council of Medical Research, India

8 figures and 21 tables, 2000

KARGER Basel · Freiburg · Paris · London · New York ·
New Delhi · Bangkok · Singapore · Tokyo · Sydney

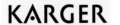

············

Artemis P. Simopoulos

4330 Klingle Street, N.W.
Washington, DC 20016 (USA)

Ramesh V. Bhat

National Institute of Nutrition
Indian Council of Medical Research
Hyderabad (India)

Library of Congress Cataloging-in-Publication Data

Street foods / volume editors, A.P. Simopoulos, R.V. Bhat
     p. cm.– (World review of nutrition and dietetics; vol. 86)
   Includes bibliographical references (p.).
   ISBN 3–8055–6927–0 (hardcover)
     1. Cookery, International. 2. Snack foods. 3. Vending stands. I. Simopoulos, Artemis
P., 1933– II. Series.

   QP141.A1 W59 vol. 86
   [TX725.A1]
   641.59–dc21

                                                                        99-026676

     Bibliographic Indices. This publication is listed in bibliographic services, including Current Contents® and Index Medicus/Medline.

     © Copyright 2000 by S. Karger AG, P.O. Box, CH–4009 Basel (Switzerland)
     www.karger.com
     Printed in Switzerland on acid-free paper by Reinhardt Druck, Basel
     ISSN 0084-2230
     ISBN 3–8055–6927–0

....
Contents

Preface

This volume on *Street Foods* provides an overview of their status in selected developed and developing countries.

The Food and Agricultural Organization of the United Nations (FAO) defines street foods as 'ready-to-eat foods and beverages prepared and/or sold by vendors and hawkers, especially in streets and other similar public places'. Street foods are a heterogeneous food category consisting of meals, drinks and snacks. They are inexpensive and available foods that, in many countries form an integral part of the diet, because they are consumed with regularity and consistency across all income groups, but particularly among the urban poor and in some countries, by children.

International organizations have paid particular attention to the safety of street foods and much less to the composition and preservation of their nutritional quality. In 1996, the World Health Organization's (WHO) Food Safety Unit Report on the essential safety requirements for street-vended foods stated that proper preparation and processing techniques are essential for ensuring the safety of street-vended foods. Three critical roles of preparation and processing were identified in the report:

(1) Preparation and processing should be adequate to eliminate or reduce hazards to an acceptable level.

(2) Preparation and processing should prevent growth of pathogens, production of toxic chemicals and the introduction of physical hazards.

(3) Preparation and processing should ensure that foods are not recontaminated.

Preparation and processing will also affect the nutritional quality of food via their influences on nutrient loss. Although fat-soluble vitamins and minerals are generally fairly stable, water-soluble vitamins are easily lost in preparation, processing, and storage. Vitamin C, thiamin, and folate are especially susceptible to being lost or destroyed.

The street food trade is large and complex. It provides an important means of generating income, particularly for women, and it is an affordable source of food for many millions of people. Therefore, street foods have been considered as a way of reducing problems of urban food insecurity and as a possible vehicle for micronutrient supplementation.

Although most of the reports have focussed mainly on developing countries, the street food trade is found in developed countries as well. Over the past 25 years, changing lifestyles have led to large numbers of people eating out. Many office workers in cities are apt to get their lunch from street vendors and many tourists in both developed and developing countries are eager to sample local fare. It is therefore timely to review the status of street foods not only from the food safety aspects, but also to examine consumption patterns and nutritional quality in selected developed and developing countries.

The authors present information on the historical aspects, profiles of street vendors and consumers, safety and nutritional quality, types of foods, snacks and drinks, and licensing.

The first paper is 'Greek street food vending: An old habit turned new' by Antonia-Leda Matalas and Mary Yannakoulia. In Greece, street foods made their appearance in the 6th Century BC with the development of urban communities. Hot lentil soup was the only available street food in the 'agora' of the Greek cities, but eating while wandering around the market was not considered appropriate. Many foods popular in ancient times were rediscovered during the Byzantine period and are popular today. The authors provide a precise evolution of the main Greek street foods from the ancient times to the present. Price is a minor factor in the selection of street foods; taste, quality and freshness are the food attributes Greeks are looking for in selecting street foods. Street foods enjoy a wide accessibility because most of the foods are not hazardous to health. The authors describe the licensing, processing, packaging and distribution of street foods. They consider street foods under these categories: (a) foods without any preparation; (b) street cooked foods, and (c) ready-to-eat foods. They provide extensive information on the nutritional, chemical and microbiological quality of street foods. The business of street foods is dominated by men. The authors conclude that street foods will hold a bigger share of the market in the future.

The next paper 'Street foods in America: a true melting pot' is by Denise Taylor and co-workers. In the USA, there is a vast array of food choices, but relatively little information about consumption patterns and their contribution to the diet of Americans. This paper provides an overview of the foods available and the health, safety and regulatory issues associated with consumption of street foods. Street foods have been part of the American scene since the 17th century. The street vendor market became a business that the lower class maintained, both as vendors and consumers. In describing the historical aspects of street foods, the authors indicate that many of the restaurant chains began as single street food stands. The types of food sold represent the ethnic groups that make up the US population today. Four cultures stand out: Italian, Mexican, Middle Eastern, and Chinese. However, many other street foods include Navajo fry bread, German bratwurst, Greek gyro and souvlaki, Indian samosas, Japanese yakitori, Caribbean roti and patties, and Argentine empanadas. The authors provide information of the nutritional quality of the street foods and discuss the microbial quality of street foods, the problems of food poisoning, the regulatory issues surrounding street foods and the profile of street vendors. Women play a minor role in street vending in the USA whereas they play a prominent role in developing countries.

The third paper 'Public (street) foods in Australia' is by Mark Wahlqvist and co-workers. They state that the concept of street foods is rarely seen as being a part of developed countries such as Australia with its 5,400 supermarkets and 130,000 other retail establishments. The preferred term is 'public foods' rather than 'street foods' since the locations of supply and consumption are more varied than the street, e.g. sports grounds, church fetes, shopping malls, cinemas. By 'public foods' they refer to the immediate purchase and consumption of ready-to-eat foods in public places. Public foods have an element of environmental proximity about them which require little anticipation, planning or preparation on the part of the consumer. They form part of the class of convenience foods but are purchased and usually consumed in a public location – though some foods are undoubtedly purchased for later consumption in the home, e.g. jams, preserved fruit and cakes from church and other fetes. They are part of a rising trend in Australian and other western societies, the convenience food trend.

The next paper 'Profile of street foods sold in Asian countries' is by Ramesh V. Bhat and Kavita Waghray. Although street foods have been around for hundreds of years, the proliferation of street foods in Asian countries is a new phenomenon. It began in the 1940s. Foods are selected because of taste and low cost, they are not selected for their nutritional value, although the food energy and protein value of cooked street food is higher than that which could be obtained from prepackaged processed food. The authors consider food safety a major issue and for this reason describe in detail the Hazard Analysis Critical Control Points (HACCP) on how to conduct the HACCP analysis in the field to determine critical control points. The HACCP concept has been applied to street foods in 23% of the countries which participated in the WHO street-vended food survey.

Drs. Bhat and Waghray continue with their paper 'Street foods in Africa'. Studies conducted in some of the African countries like Nigeria and Morocco have shown that the major street food vendors usually earn more than the country's minimum wage. In Nigeria it is cheaper to buy street food than to cook it. Eating street foods begins in infancy. In Senegal, yogurt is frequently given to the babies as weaning food and is never prepared at home. Street foods were the major source of nutrients for many of the adolescents (n = 142) in Abeokuta (Nigeria). Between 40 and 70% intake of all the major sources of food groups were obtained from street foods which were the major source of dairy products (70%), legumes (60%), fish (50%), meat (50%) and eggs (50%); 21% of energy for males and 29% energy for females was supplied by street foods. Street foods also supplied greater than 50% total proteins, 64% calcium and 60% vitamin A for both males and females. For other minerals (iron) and vitamins (thiamine and ascorbic acid) street foods supplied greater than 50% of total intake. Selection of street foods is based on taste, price, and last on nutritional quality.

Drs. Bhat and Waghray also examine 'Street foods in Latin America' in the next paper. Street food industry is part of the informal economy of the Latin American countries. Most of the street vendors earn more than the minimum wage.

Miriam de Chavez and co-workers look specifically at Mexican street food in 'The sale of street food in Latin America. The Mexican case: Joy or jeopardy?' in the paper which follows. Mexico has an old tradition of street foods. Fruits and juices are prominent items along with cooked snacks and meals. As in other Latin American countries, food safety and licensing are important issues, as are the economic aspects of street foods which represent an important sector of the economy.

Liora Gvion-Rosenberg and Naomi Trostler describe 'Street food vending: The Israeli scenario' in the final paper. Street food vending as seen in developing countries is not part of the Israeli gastronomic scene. The Israeli version of street foods is generally available at kiosks and small shops. Falafel, sunflower seeds, nuts, ice cream or pizza are all part of the daily culinary street scene. Israeli food fairs are also described. The nature of the Israeli trend in street foods includes two major characteristics. First, it is an established and organized activity, mainly localized in commercial urban centers. Second, it is mainly for snacking purposes, and does not conform to the FAO definition because it is neither prepared nor sold by street vendors and hawkers.

This volume should be of interest to scientists and policy makers in the area of international health, nutrition, food and trade; and to physicians, nutritionists, dieticians, food scientists, anthropologists, sociologists and directors of public health departments.

Artemis P. Simopoulos, MD

Simopoulos AP, Bhat RV (eds): Street Foods.
World Rev Nutr Diet. Basel, Karger, 2000, vol 86, pp 1–24

....

Greek Street Food Vending: An Old Habit Turned New

Antonia-Leda Matalas, Mary Yannakoulia

Department of Nutrition and Dietetics, Harokopio University, Athens, Greece

Everyday life in modern Greek cities involves long working hours and increased commuting time. The amount of time devoted to the acquisition, preparation, and even consumption of food has declined. Additionally, a substantial breakfast does not constitute a familiar practice for most of the inhabitants of Greek cities [1, 2]. In such a situation, both traditional street foods and items produced by the fast-food industry, foods characterized by high palatability and availability, and low prices, offer convenient meal alternatives or snacks.

Selling and bartering goods in a nonsettled manner was one of the first commercial activities man undertook since prehistoric times. In the modern era the basic food procurement techniques humans practiced, namely hunting, gathering, animal raising, and horticulture are largely abandoned; food is mostly attained through commerce, and highly structured activities for trading goods have developed. Small-scale vending by nonsettled traders and peddling have been observed to decline spontaneously whenever a society reached a certain stage of economic development. In the various regions of Western Europe peddlers disappeared during the 18th and 19th centuries [3]. Braudel [3] states, however, that there was a revival of this archaic form of trade in the suburbs of industrial towns poorly served by the ordinary distribution networks. The practice of supplying ready-for-consumption food in public places must have appeared as a necessity with the segregation of large populations within urban settings who have limited time and facilities to prepare food during working hours. This latter type of food vending became characteristic of everyday life in 20th century urban centers.

The nutritional and socioeconomic roles of street foods in developing countries as well as in Europe and North America have attracted a great deal of interest during the last decade. During the past four decades street food consumption in Greek urban centers has apparently increased, as a result of an accelerated migration from rural areas to the towns and cities [4]. To the best of our knowledge, this is the first published work that examines the use of street foods and their impact in the life of people in Greece.

A definition of street foods in a 'Greek perspective' will be attempted, with regard to their present situation, the role, and the needs they currently meet. In this context, the term 'street food' describes a wide range of foods, sold – and sometimes prepared – from mobile carts, fixed stands or shops in the street, the latter having a more permanent structure, without or with limited seating facilities. They are easily accessible from the street, even when the vendors' stalls/mini shops are not located outdoors. These foods are consumed as purchased without requiring use of cutlery or any further preparation and processing. An innovation has been observed recently in Greece and some of the traditional street foods have been included in the product lists of fast-food chains. This is part of a tendency in the Greek fast-food industry to expand its realm to ethnic cuisines, including traditional Greek, Cypriot, Chinese, and Mexican [5]. The American-style ones, such as hamburgers, pizzas and french fries, as well as other types of fast-foods consumed in Greece are not considered 'street foods' and therefore will not be examined in this paper. In the first part, the historical perspective of Greek street foods will be discussed, and in the second part their current status will be investigated.

Methods

Literature search was conducted to reveal the origins of Greek street foods. Although the bibliography is rich in data regarding the use of street foods in past times, information on their current role in Greece is scarce. Much of the material presented in this paper has been collected through interviews with people involved in the street food sector, including vendors, manufacturers, administrative officers and consumers. The interviews sought information on first appearance of street foods in modern Greek cities, recipes and methods of preparation, acquisition of raw materials, size of production, prices, health safety issues, pertinent legislation, and consumption patterns. The nutrient content of Greek street foods was derived from recipes provided by manufacturers and vendors, with the assistance of the UK Food Composition Tables [6] and published data on the composition of Greek foods [7, 8].

Historical Perspective of Greek Street Foods

Cities in Greece with urban characteristics appear as early as the 6th century BC. Literature sources, such as theatrical plays and historical accounts, have passed down to us information on the structure and commercial activities of the Athenian and other food markets, the *agoras*, in classical times [9].[1] The economy of the Athenian city was based on agriculture and the life of the town was integrated with that of the surrounding countryside [3]. In the Athenian *agora*, farmers were one of its most vivid components, selling from their stands in the street a variety of products: wheat and barley, freshly made *koulouri* (described below), vegetables, fruits, fish and seafood, poultry, preserved meat, dairy, wine and vinegar, nuts and sweets [9, 11, 12]. Albeit a prevailing urban character, street vending in classical Athens never really expanded to ready-for-consumption foods. The only mention of food served in the street refers to hot lentil soup that was available in the market [13]. Theophrastos provides us with evidence that ancient Athenians disapproved of eating an item that was just purchased while wandering around the market [14].

At least two modern street foods can be traced to antiquity, the koulouri and the cheese pie [12, 15]. The κολλύριο (kollyrio),[2] as the koulouri was known in ancient times, was a small-sized, round-shaped bread made of barley flour. It was consumed mainly by children. The kollyrio of the ancient Greeks reappears in the Byzantine period, under the names of *kollykio* and *semiti*.[3] All three terms, koulouri, kollyrio, and kollykio share a common etymological origin, implying a type of small and roundish bread [18] while the Byzantine term semiti has been derived from the Greek word for semolina, *semigdali*. The term πλακούντας τυρόνωτος (cheese pie) is mentioned in ancient Greek literature, namely in theatrical dialogues, providing evidence that this foodstuff was known by ancient Greeks [15, 19].

Because many of the street foods sold in Greece today were introduced to the Greek mainland from Constantinople and Asia Minor during the past 150 years, the study of street food vending in Constantinople and Smyrna, a major commerical center in Asia Minor, sheds light on our understanding of its contemporary situation in Greece.

Street food vending was a prominent feature of everday life in Constantinople. A number of Greek authors give details on types of street foods available and the profile of street food vendors frequenting its markets. Constantinople

[1] The city-state of Athens hosted in the fifth century BC 180,000 Athenian citizens, women, and children (half of them *metikoi*), and some 150,000–160,000 slaves and freedmen [10].

[2] The term 'collyrium' used in ophthalmology was derived from the Greek word 'κολλύριο' (small round bread) and denotes the practice of using a piece of soft bread soaked in various remedies as an eye compress [16].

[3] As mentioned by the Byzantine historian Porphyrogenitos, a small ring-shaped bread was sold in Constantinople in 9th century [17].

was a major urban center of the Byzantine and Ottoman empires, largely populated by Greeks.[4] After the 1600s, Constantinople emerged into a multinational metropolis, attracting immigrants from even remote territories of the Ottoman empire [20]. Mobile street vendors, known as 'the round-about professionals' (επαγγελματίες του γύρου), represented an important group of food traders in Constantinople [21–23]. At that time they had not founded yet their own professional associations, but were organized under the auspices of professional associations that represented the particular product they were trading [22]. Among professionals involved in food trading, Greeks and Armenians were represented by the largest numbers [23]. The koulouri, the cheese pie,[5] the *boyatsa* (type of custard pie), the *chalvas* (honey cake), baked carrots and coffee were the most common food items offered by mobile vendors during the 17th and 18th centuries [22]. It is worth mentioning that vendors were strictly specializing in one item only, an attribute that is retained till today in Greek cities.

During the 19th and early 20th centuries, the variety of street foods appearing in Constantinople expanded. More than fifteen different types of street foods could be identified: semiti (also called *sesamato*), *kanavosesamato* (a variety of semiti), cheese pie, boyatsa, meat pie (*boureki*), pilaf, fried liver, fried meatballs (*keftes*), fried bonito fish,[6] roasted chick peas (*strayalia*), a type of popcorn (*misirbouida*) and boiled corn-on-the-cob [21–23]. Cheese pies and boyatsa were always made with sheep butter. These items were prepared by specialized bakeries that were not licensed to make or sell bread [23]. While most of the foods sold in the street were preprepared, some items were, at least partly, prepared upon the client's order. Interesting is the case of the so-called *arnaout-tzieri*, a type of sandwich that consisted of a quarter of a bread loaf stuffed with fried liver (*tzieri*), chopped parsley and onion, while white beans could also be added depending on the client's wish [23]. In the food market of Athens today, one can still buy a similar type of sandwich made with fried liver [25]. A large variety of sweets and candies were also sold by mobile vendors during the same time period, including a sesame dessert (*pastelli*), walnut cake (*karythato*), honey cake (*chalvas*), 'triangle' or *trigono*, a

---

[4] Constantinople was the original name of Istanbul, a metropolitan city located in the European territory of today's Turkey. Constantinople, established by the Emperor Constantine in 330 AD at the site of the old Greek city Byzantium, was the capital of the Byzantine Empire until 1453 when it was captured by the Ottoman Turks.

[5] The Byzantine cheese pie was called 'αρτοτυρίτης πλακούντας', a term that can be translated to 'Cheese-bread placenta'.

[6] According to Rice [24], in Constantinople of Medieval times, fishermen were forbidden to sell raw fish (in order to avoid low prices); they were however allowed to sell cooked fish. This practice may have led to the appearance of cooked fish as a street food.

delicacy made of phyllo dough, milk and honey, shaped into small triangles, and candy-floss (*malli grias*) [21, 23]. Greek sailors, when in harbor in Constantinople or the neighboring harbors, used to indulge on delicacies available in this great city. A 19th century nautical document provides evidence that, in contrast with the harbor of Constantinople, boyatsa and chalvas were not available in harbors of the Greek mainland and Aegean Sea [26].

Not only foods, but also hot beverages were sold by mobile vendors in Constantinople. The most common among them was the salepi, prepared by boiling the root of the plant *Orchis mascula* (salepi) and infiltrating the juice with the aid of a special apparatus that all respective street vendors had on their small carriage. Wandering coffee vendors, carrying cups of coffee on the traditional tray, could also be seen in the markets of Constantinople [23]. Vendors were named after the particular item they were trading. The vendor of semiti was named *semitzis*; of boyatsa, *boyatsatzis*; of tzieri, *tziertzis*; of salepi, *salepitzis*, and so on.

Smyrna, a city founded by the Greeks in 1100 BC, had in the early 19th century the world's largest Greek population. The city of Smyrna, on the Asia Minor coast, also became an international center after 1800s and experienced a great cultural influence from Western European countries [27]. The Western influence exhibited itself in types and names of street foods available. Ice cream was sold by mobile vendors in the streets of the city during the 19th and early 20th centuries, and it was called *glashato*, after the French word for ice cream, *glace*, while respective vendors were known as *glashatzides* [28]. By contrast, in Constantinople the Turkish word for ice cream, *doudourma*, was used and vendors were called *doudourmatzides* [22]. Roasted chestnuts and sugar-glazed red apples were also sold in the streets, along with various types of sherbets, including the traditional salepi, and a sweet almond drink, the *soumada*, introduced to Smyrna from the Greek island of Chios [28]. Other hot beverages known to be sold in Smyrna in the late 18th and 19th centuries were tea, sage, dittany, and cinnamon-flavored drinks [28]. Furthermore, most of the street foods mentioned above to be consumed in Constantinople were also available in Smyrna.

The cities of the Greek mainland, including the modern city of Athens, gained importance as urban centers during the second half of the 19th century.[7] Street foods available in the streets of the Greek capital in the mid-1800s, koulouri, cheese pies and boyatsa, ice cream, sherbets, chalvas, roasted chick peas, chestnuts and salepi, were introduced as such from Constantinople and Smyrna [30–32]. Street foods vendors in Athens marked its everyday life. The appearance of a salepi vendor became synonymous to an early morning hour

---

[7] In 1837, Athenians numbered to 15,000 only [29].

('to wake up with the first salepi') [31, 33]. Numerous photos and drawings depicting the picturesque early street food vendors have been published and constitute a major part of the evidence we have in appearance of street food items [32, 34, 35]. When Athens grew in size after 1920 and hosted large numbers of visitors and immigrants, the first taverns appeared selling dishes to be eaten by the clients while standing [36]. These foods can be viewed as types of street foods.

Souvlaki and gyros were introduced in Athens after World War II. In the 1950s, cooks who immigrated from Asia Minor and the Middle East started preparing and selling gyros in the Greek capital. As a street food, gyros preceded the well-known souvlaki both in Athens and in most Greek cities and towns. Although souvlaki can be traced back to the 19th century,[8] it was lauched as a street food only in late 1960s, by businessmen of the Boeotia region [pers. commun., Mr. Xenophon Tsiboyannis, a 60-year-old cook specialized in gyros preparation and cooking].

Not all street foods found in Constantinople were reproduced in the Greek mainland, probably due to the fact that Athens and other cities did not reach the importance of Constantinople as a commercial center. In addition, legislative actions taken by the government during the past 15 years have contributed to the disappearance of several traditional street foods [38]. The pertinent legislation, aiming at improving public health, clearly states which types of foods can be distributed by street vendors, and forbids items such as nonstandardized ice creams, chocolate products, candies and beverages.

The appearance of items domesticated in the New World among Greek street foods deserves a comment. Corn, peanuts, sunflower seeds and tomato (as part of the pita bread souvlaki) were integrated into Greek street food vending only in the 20th century. During the past 30 years, roasted corn-on-the-cob is sold by street vendors in towns and cities specially during the evening hours in summer months (fig. 1). The corn vendors, much like the chestnut vendors, settle their stalls at specific sites determined by the local municipality. The freshly roasted corn-on-the-cob is particularly popular among children, but is also consumed by adults. It is worth mentioning that this is the only way Greeks have prepared corn as a food until recently. Otherwise, corn has been cultivated in Greece mainly for animal feeding. Some canned corn, often imported, is used in salads, but its use is mainly limited to salads offered at American-type fast food facilities and some other restaurants.

---

[8] Gustave Flaubert, in 1850, during a visit to the Greek countryside in Boeotia wrote that the Greeks were grilling pieces of meat on a bamboo stick [37].

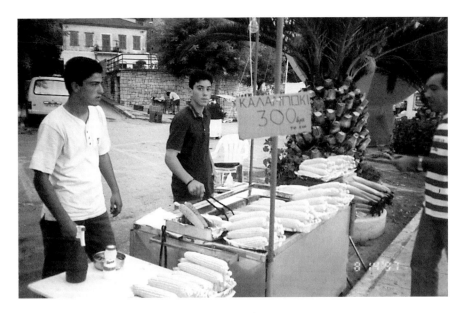

Fig. 1. Street vendors selling corn-on-the-cob.

The Main Greek Street Foods

Among the various types of street foods available in Greek cities, the souvlaki, the *gyros*, the *koulouri* and the several types of dairy pies are the ones most frequently consumed. The souvlaki and the gyros (table 1) are sold by special mini shops with limited or no seating facilities. They can be eaten as such as as a filling in a rolled-up pita bread together with tomato pieces, chopped onions, and small quantities of *tzatziki* (yogurt dip with cucumber and garlic). The Greek word *souvlaki* means small skewer, but in everyday use it implies pieces of meat served on the skewer. Often referred to as *kalamaki*, a word derived from the bamboo sticks that were used originally, the souvlaki is grilled on charcoals and is served sprinkled with salt and oregano. Its average size is 40 g, consisting of 5–6 pork cubes, one of which is usually pure pork fat added to enhance flavor (fig. 2). Similar skewers of small chunks of various types of meats are also eaten in other parts of the world, such as in Indonesia and Bagladesh in Southeast Asia, and in Senegal in Africa [39]. The Greek gyros is one of the best known Greek foods worldwide. Meaning 'round or circle', its name was derived from a unique preparation method: the meat is placed around a long vertical metal skewer and is cooked while it rotates at a slow pace in front of a vertical grill (fig. 3). The meat usually weighs, as a

Table 1. Description and methods of preparation for the main Greek street foods

Street food	Description/method of preparation
Boyatsa	milk dessert made with flaky pastry and custard filling; topped with fine sugar
Tyropita/spanakopita (cheese/spinach pie)	flaky pastry or phyllo dough and cheese filling (traditionally feta or telemes cheese)
Kastana/kalampokia (chestnuts/corn-on-the-cob)	grilled on the charcoals
Koulouri	small ring-shaped bread covered with sesame seeds
Loukoumas	ring-shaped fried dough sprinkled with sugar
Malli grias	candy floss
Ksiroi karpoi (nuts and seeds)	roasted and salted pistachios, peanuts, chick peas, sunflower seeds
Passatempo	roasted and salted pumpkin seeds
Pastelli	sesame seeds covered with honey
Pita sandwich	
Pita bread	round flat dough made of flour, yeast and salt, used for souvlaki covering
Souvlaki	grilled pork meat cubes (serving size: approximately 40 g)
Gyros	slices of grilled spiced meat, pork or beef (serving size: approximately 40 g)

whole, about 20 kg, from which small slices are cut upon order. In Middle Eastern countries, gyros is traditionally made of lamb or beef, as pork is a food prohibited to Muslims. In Greece, however, it is mostly made of pork or beef meat heavily spiced and is available in two types. One type, the *doner kebab*[9] or simply *doner*, is prepared from ground beef and/or lamb meat shaped into a cone around the vertical skewer. This is the type commonly seen in Turkey. The second type comprises slices of pork meat put together on the skewer, and bears similarities with the Middle Eastern *shwarma*, which is made of lamb. This kind of gyros emerged in Greece in the early 1970s, after the prohibition of the usage of ground meat and the enforcement of using pork meat in gyros. Two decades afterwards, the ground meat prohibition was withdrawn; however the largest portion of all gyros sold in Greece today is made of pork meat [pers. commun. with officers of the Greek Health Department].

[9] Doner means 'to turn' in Turkish, while kebab means 'meat' in Arabic [16, 40].

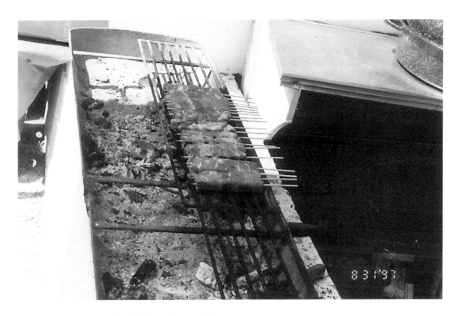

Fig. 2. Souvlaki grilled on charcoals.

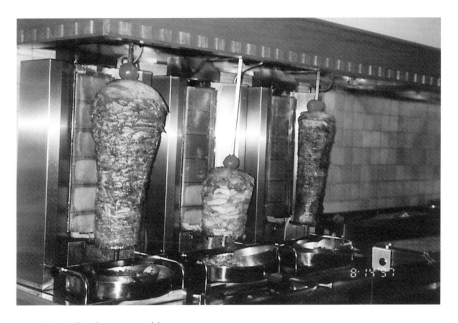

Fig. 3. Greek gyros cooking.

The 'pita-bread sandwich' made with either souvlaki or gyros bears a lot of similarities with other 'finger-foods', i.e. hot dogs, hamburgers, tacos, and sandwiches. Breads such as pitas in Greece and the Middle East, buns and baguettes in Europe and US, chapattis and pooris in India and tortillas in Mexico are used in lieu of utensils [41]. The basic idea is grabbing the food with one's fingers, without the need of cutlery. In contrast with the wide use the pita bread finds in other cultures in accompanying meals, in Greece it finds no other uses than enveloping souvlaki and gyros. New recipes of the 'pita bread sandwich' have been lately introduced allowing for the addition of new relishes, such as french fries, tomato sauce, and green pepper, while gyros made of chicken is also available in few outlets. No vegetarian version, however, has been launched so far in Greece.[10]

The *koulouri* (table 1) bears a time-lasting quality, being popular among Greeks of all ages since ancient times. To this day, this ring-shaped bread is sold by specialized vendors, stationary or mobile, who cluster in major downtown commercial and public services areas, markets and crossroads. During the past couple of years, one can observe the phenomenon of ambulatory street vendors around traffic lights of main arteries selling *koulouria* to daily commuters, providing a king of 'drive-in' service, so that drivers do not have to get out of their cars (fig. 4).

Dairy pies, specifically cheese pie, spinach pie and *boyatsa* (custard pie) (table 1), constitute the breakfast of choice for a large number of Greeks. They are available in every neighborhood, sold by mobile vendors, bakeries and specialized mini shops. Greeks usually consume them on their way to or at work.

Consumption and availability of these 'core' street foods exhibit a diurnal pattern that follows people's activities and food habits. During the morning hours freshly made koulouri and pies are available. Data collected during a national survey in the 1980s reveal that 44% of Greek men and 32% of Greek women eat cheese pie, koulouri or sandwich as a midday snack at least once a week (from which 36 and 22%, respectively, have these items more than four times a week) [1]. Pies are available till early afternoon, while koulouri vendors close down their stands around noon. From noon till late in the evening, people prefer souvlaki and gyros. A considerable number of vendors operate throughout the night, offering souvlaki, along with the more recently introduced hot dog sandwiches, to youngsters after late-night entertainment. People have thus the opportunity to eat street foods all day and night and are no longer confined to traditional mealtimes.

---

[10] A great variety of sandwiches made with pita bread, including some vegetarian types, are part of the traditional cuisine in Middle-Eastern countries [42].

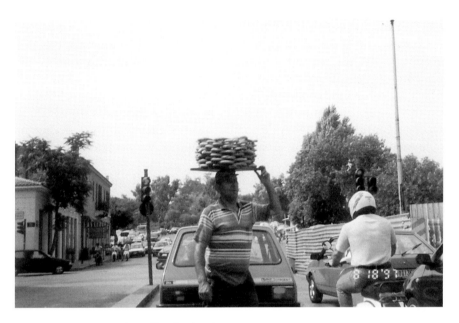

Fig. 4. Street vendor selling koulouria to commuters.

A great deal of 'secondary' street foods are typical of particular seasons or special occasions and events, complementing the ever-present souvlaki. Roasted nuts, pulses, seeds (pistachios, peanuts, chick peas, pumpkin seeds or *passatempo,*[11] sunflower seeds) and raisins are eaten during leisure time. In festivals and sports events, and predominantly when these take place during the summer in open-air sites, many hawkers can be spotted at the entrance selling nuts and raisins. Chestnuts and corn-on-the-cob, grilled on charcoals in the streets, are popular items during winter and summer months, respectively. Some sweetened foods are also sold by street vendors, namely *loukoumas* (a type of doughnut), *malli grias* (candy floss) and *pastelli* (sesame dessert) (table 1). Candy floss is hardly found nowadays anywhere else apart from amusement parks, where the few remaining vendors puff to young visitors their sweet delicacy. Ice cream and traditional beverages, items that had a widespread use as street foods during past decades, nowadays are only found in historic markets and tend to disappear.

Selling sites of street foods are determined by the clientele and the type of food sold. Although vendors cluster in market areas of big cities, they are not restricted there and can be found in every site where there is a target

[11] The term passatempo means 'to pass the time'.

group of consumers. Those with mobile carts can move according to demand, for example to areas with high tourist concentrations in summer months. Vacation resorts are frequented by numerous street vendors, and tourists can taste corn-on-the-cob grilled on charcoals and nuts. It has been shown that an increase in fast food consumption is noted during summertime and holidays [43] and, though no data exist on street foods, it is reasonable to conclude that their consumption follows a similar trend. Concomitantly, a decline in koulouri demand occurs in urban centers during the summer months, as reported by street vendors.

Greek street foods are primarily based on wheat and enriched with seeds (as sesame in koulouri), cheese, fat, vegetables, or pieces of meat. Notably, street foods do not include any fish or seafood. This fact exemplifies the dominating role of wheat flour and bread as staple foods in the Greek diet since classical times [44, 45]. Foods sold in the streets fulfill the criteria of inexpensive filling items, high in calories but lack social function and prestige [46]. The qualities of street foods can be contrasted with those of the traditional Greek 'meze', an assortment of small pieces of several types of food eaten between meals and served with distilled liquors (ouzo and raki). The 'meze' is served at *kafenio* (traditional coffee shops) or special ouzo shops at street sidewalks. However, the 'meze' does not possess any 'filling' quality and, unlike street foods, is eaten around the table, having as its main purpose to facilitate social interaction with table companions and to accompany one's drink [47]. Made from a large variety of foods, including fish and seafood, cheese, delicatessen type meats, vegetables and pickles, the Greek 'meze' is clearly differentiated from local street foods [48].

Profile of Street Food Vendors

Numbers

It is difficult to estimate the actual number of street food vendors in Greek cities, as many of them operate illegally. Existing official statistics based on registered vendors, greatly underestimate both the stationary and the ambulatory ones. Although the official license is a prerequisite for the legal operation of both types [49], only 77 of the stationary food vendors in Athens are equipped with one. Half of them have a license for selling koulouri, i.e. 38 vendors, a number that represents no more than a third of the active koulouri vendors in Athens. Another 44% of the registered vendors are licensed to sell either corn-on-the-cob or chestnuts at designated sites and only 6% sell nuts and raisins [Municipality of Athens, unpubl. data].

Licensing

License supply used to be the responsibility of the General Commissioner of Police, whereas since 1970, street food vendors are under the control of municipality and prefecture authorities. Municipality authorities have set a fixed number of licenses to allocate to stationary street food vendors, a number that has remained unchanged over the past few decades despite an increasing demand. Criteria used for license provision put emphasis on social status and special consideration is given to disadvantaged people, such as the handicapped, war victims, and persons having more than three children. Additionally the applicant or the holder should provide official evidence that his or her annual earnings are below a certain threshold designated to approximate the minimum wage earning in order to be eligible for a 'site'. All site occupants are obliged to provide a moderate annual fee to the municipality.

Gender

In Greece, street food enterprise represents a business that is dominated by men, and the role of women is only supportive, as evidenced by official data as well as by the authors' experiences. Street food vending in Greece differs significantly from that in developing countries, where the woman's role is prominent in all stages of preparation and distribution [39, 50]. In these countries, women cook the foods they sell in the street themselves thus promoting their own products [51, 52]. The limited role of women in Greece can be attributed to a legislative regulation designating that no home-prepared foods can be distributed by street vendors. When street cooking is required, such as is the case for souvlaki, roasted chestnuts and corns-on-the-cob sold by street vendors, cooking techniques employed are confined to barbecuing, a mode of preparation that in western cultures is associated with the male gender.

Socioeconomic Aspects of Street Foods

Representing low-cost foods and meal substitutes, street foods have a modest share in the overall food expenses of Greek households. Data from the latest Household Budget Survey (1993–1994) reveal that the consumption of street foods is a predominantly urban characteristic, being now more prevalent in the two main Greek cities, Athens and Thessaloniki [53]. Amounts of money spent per capita for street food purchases in the various rural and semi-urban areas are half or even less of that spent in either Athens or Thessaloniki, a difference due to the decrease in demand in smaller cities and towns.

Consumption of individual street foods in Greece has never been addressed by food consumption surveys, and therefore, can only be indirectly evaluated. Based on information collected among koulouri bakers and vendors, we estimated that around 40,000–50,000 koulouri pieces are sold daily in the streets of the Greek capital. Koulouri consumption, however, has declined by 50% during the last decade, as evidenced by a reported decrease in production rates. Youngsters in particular seem to increasingly prefer other types of quickly consumed items, such as croissants, sandwiches, and various fast foods. Consumption of fast foods between 1993 and 1996 has markedly increased by 100% [43].

Unlike the koulouri, souvlaki and gyros seem to maintain their prestige among members of all age groups and social classes [43]. In the form of a pita sandwich, souvlaki and gyros represent complex foods and possess a hedonic character, qualities that enhance status and prestige [54]. Data taken from pita manufacturers show that, in the whole country, 800,000 pita sandwiches are consumed on a daily basis, i.e. every day one out of every ten Greeks consumes a pita sandwich either as a street food or at shops with some sitting facilities. Furthermore, there is a considerable number of souvlaki eaten without the pita, as a more convenient and cheap alternative. Although pita sandwich is popular among all sexes and socioeconomic groups, a class gradient can be observed. As one moves to areas accommodating lower socioeconomic groups, the number of souvlaki and gyros shops is increasing and people prefer larger pita sandwiches, made with bigger pita and abundant relishes [pers. commun. Mr. Kostas Yannopoulos, director of a large pita bread company].

Regular street food consumers are people who work in downtown areas, as well as people that habitually stay away from home for long hours, such as students and shoppers. Factors associated with street food consumption include socioeconomic status, educational level, income, and age. Street foods are characteristically inexpensive items. Literature provides evidence that in developing countries consumption of street foods is associated with low socioeconomic status. Discussing the situation in these countries, Solomons [55] has argued that 'fast food restaurants of the urban poor around the world are the mobile carts of street food vendors, and street foods are the fare of the urban working class'. In Greece, however, impact of various factors influencing selection of street foods has never been assessed. A recent study that assessed the consumers' food-related behavior in Europe, showed that price was a minor factor in determining food choices of Greek respondents, in sharp contrast with the dominant role attributes such as taste, quality, and freshness exhibited [56]. According to the same study, among all Europeans, Greeks are the most influenced by family food preferences, a finding that reconfirms the importance of traditional habits in shaping food patterns. In that line, Greek street foods have a long tradition behind them and enjoy a widespread acceptability. In addition, they represent food items that are devoid of the stigma of health hazard.

Economics

Undoubtedly, the street food sector is an important provider of income for many members of urban communities [57]. Production and distribution of street foods provide employment and contribute to the overall urban economy. This sector offers appreciable advantages: enterprises are relatively small in size, require low start-up capital, minor investment in facilities, while they allow for family-run businesses. As there is no competitive pricing, earnings depend exclusively on clientele size, and usually rank above average wage. The possibility of earning relatively high incomes along with a low capital investment (initial nonrecurring expenditure) has attracted a great number of vendors. That is the reason for having so many ambulatory street food vendors. The majority of them are low-skilled professionals, who work under an illegal status, and have an opportunistic relationship with street vending, while a significant percentage of them are immigrants.

Processing, Distribution and Packaging of Street Foods

For practical purposes, street foods can be classified according to the processing/preparation they require [58]: (a) foods without any preparation, (b) street-cooked foods, and (c) ready-to-eat foods.

Street foods belonging to the first category cannot be seen in Greece. All street foods sold in this country undergo at least a minor stage of preparation. It is the necessity of cooking, a cultural transformation, to turn produce from the field into food. This 'cookedness' can be observed in all aspects of eating behavior and constitutes an overall quality of Greek eating patterns: no food item is consumed in its 'natural' state, apart from that picked in the field and eaten on the spot [59]. Thus, some street foods, such as koulouri and dairy pies, are preprepared and ready-to-eat, while others, such as chestnuts, souvlaki and gyros, are cooked on site and sometimes prepared upon client's order. Most of them are produced on a daily basis and consumed freshly made, with the exception of nuts that are roasted in big lots. Freshness, and even warmth, are essential qualities of street foods.[12]

---

[12] Unsold koulouri are always discarded or used as animal feed. However, sometimes unsold cheese pies, gyros, and cooked souvlaki, are preserved and reheated next day.

The specialization of producers to a particular item is not a recent advancement; even in Byzantine times, most street foods were massively produced by small-scale factories, which, had to fulfill legal requirements [23]. Today, the koulouri demand in the greater area of Athens is met by only 3–4 specialized bakeries that supply all street koulouri vendors. The same basic pattern also holds for other types of street foods. Few specialized bakeries produce a great part of the cheese pies and boyatsa consumed, around fifty factories supply pita bread to all parts of Greece and there are butcheries that prepare souvlaki and gyros skewers for the provision of the corresponding mini shops [pers. commun. with vendors].

Nutritional Value

Koulouri

The Greek koulouri is basically a bread substitute, and has a comparable nutritional value. Its nutrient content was estimated based on a recipe provided by specialized bakers, with the use of the UK Food Composition Tables [6]. Koulouri is made of white flour, water and yeast, with the addition of sugar, small quantities of vegetable oil, and salt, and, after baking, it is sprinkled with sesame seeds. An average koulouri weighs approximately 40 g and provides 90–100 kcal, of which 70% is derived from carbohydrate. Although it does not constitute an important source of any essential nutrient, it provides small quantities of unsaturated fats and vitamin E, a significant part of which come from the sesame seeds. Koulouri can be regarded as a carbohydrate-rich snack, supplementing the quick breakfast of Greeks. Compared to other foods commonly eaten as snacks, such as cookies, chocolate bars, donuts and croissants, it provides less fat and, most importantly, is free from fatty acids of questionable quality, i.e. trans-fatty acids, and certain types of saturated fats.

Pies

Cheese and other types of pies are made with flaky pastry or phyllo dough and various types of filling, usually a mix consisting of cheese, spinach or custard. Dough and pastries used are prepared with generous amounts of margarine and/or animal fat, resulting in a ready-to-eat food that is rich in saturated and trans-fatty acids. A chemical analysis of local Greek foods that was done in Australia, showed that cheese and spinach pie have a high fat content and a P/M/S ratio of 0.3/0.6/1 and 0.4/0.6/1, respectively [7]. Fatty acid analysis of spinach has shown that ω-3 fatty acids appear at levels of 0.89 mg/g wet weight, so we presume that, although not generously, spinach

Table 2. Macronutrient content and relative prices of the Greek pita sandwich and the American hamburger

Food	Weight (g)	Energy content (kcal)	Percent energy derived from			Price[3]/weight (drachmas/g)	Price[3]/kcal (drachmas/kcal)
			protein	CHO	fat		
Cheeseburger[1]	115	307	20	41	39	3.9	1.5
Pita sandwich with souvlaki or gyros[2]	ca. 180	360	ca. 20	ca. 40	ca. 40	ca. 1.6	ca. 0.8

[1] Data taken from Paige [60] (Source: McDonalds Corporation).
[2] Due to absence of a standardized recipe and method of preparation, values of macronutrient content vary.
[3] Indicative prices used: cheeseburger: 450 drs/piece (range 400–500 drs); pita sandwich: 300 drs/piece (range: 280–320 drs).

pie, if eaten on a daily basis, may contribute to the overall ω-3 fatty acids intake [8]. Regarding its mineral content, cheese pie contains 140–200 mg Ca/ 100 g, a value that classifies it among the high calcium foods.

Pita Sandwiches/Souvlaki and Gyros

The pita sandwiches made with souvlaki or gyros are high calorie foods providing 340–390 kcal per serving. Average souvlaki weighs 180 g of which 15–20 g are fat, providing 37–44% of total calories depending on whether the pita is sauté in vegetable oil or plain grilled. It also qualifies for a good source of high quality protein and thiamin, providing approximately 19 g and 0.5 mg per serving, respectively. The souvlaki supplies appreciable quantities of calcium, iron, zinc and potassium, but is a poor source of dietary fiber and vitamin C. Salt is usually used in abundance in most stages of preparation, hence the sodium content of the pita sandwiches is high.

The pita sandwich has a macro-nutrient profile similar to that of its fast food counterpart, the hamburger (table 2). Both the pita sandwich and the hamburger are foods rich in fat, containing 40% of total calories as fat. Ramifications, however, can be noticed in regards with aspects not related to nutritional value. Hamburger is a standardized and massively produced food item, meaning that all production and distribution parameters are kept rigorously stable. Cost and other considerations lead to a minimalistic in nature product, as everything is reduced to its sparest, most utilitarian form [41]. The Greek pita sandwich, on the other hand, fulfills the attributes of handmade products: the composition of each sandwich purchased depends on a multitude of factors, notwithstanding the mood of vendor and chance. It is a much larger finger-food than the hamburger and, although inexpensive, it does not constitute a cheap or junk food. To the Greek consumer, the pita sandwich represents a food of a better cost-to-nutrient ratio (table 2). Lastly, one should not forget that eating a pita sandwich involves a risk of spilling drips of garlicky yogurt on one's clothes. A similar event is unlikely to happen while devouring a hamburger.

The Secondary Greek Street Foods: Nuts, Pulses, Seeds, Raisins, Corn and Chestnuts

As street foods, nuts, pulses and seeds are eaten seasonally or on special occasions, but thanks to their role in traditional Greek culinary habits they represent important components of the typical Greek diet [61]. Nuts constitute notably nutrient-dense foods. Despite a great variety, the various types of nuts have in common some basic characteristics. Firstly, energy content is high due to the relatively high fat content. Indicatively, a small packet of pictachios (45 g, weighed with shells) contains approximately 150 kcal and 14 g of fat, while a small packet of peanuts (60 g) contains 300 kcal and 27 g of fat [6]. Most nuts contain generous amounts of monounsaturated fatty acids and fiber, while walnuts are a rich source of ω-3 fatty acids [62]. They also supply important amounts of vitamin E, folic acid, vitamins B_1 and B_6, magnesium, iron, zinc, copper and manganese [6, 63].

Among the goods the nut-sellers offer, roasted chick peas and dried raisins, items that have a long history in Greek street food vending, are always present. These foods are of high carbohydrate content and lower caloric value than the nuts. Their nutritional merit stems from a high potassium and low sodium content, as well as from the appreciable mineral and vitamin amounts they contain [6].

Chestnuts and corn are also foods rich in carbohydrates, with a low total and saturated fat content. Chestnuts are rich in fiber, potassium and iron. Sweet corn is characterized by a high carotenoid content, and is particularly rich in zeaxanthin and β-cryptoxanthin. Vitamin A values of the sweet corn cultivars were found to range from 5.0–7.7 RE per 100 g [64].

Regulation of Street Food Vending

Relevant legislation on street food vending covers most of the areas of interest: license acquisition, sanitary control, types of items sold by food hawkers, preparation of foods and methods of distribution. Current legislation regarding sanitary conditions and suitability of food items was enacted in 1984 [38]. Price control used to be a measure to limit arbitrary pricing, but since 1992, street food vendors operate in a free economy market [pers. commun., Helene Mavrouka, officer of the Greek Ministry of Internal Affairs].

Since 1983, in an attempt to legalize and control street food vending, the Greek government requires that all vendors hold official operation licenses. Despite a detailed legislation, the Greek state is far from controlling street food vendors, and as mentioned above, a large number of outdoor hawkers operate illegally. The restricted number of available licensed sites, along with the bureaucratic procedures, discourage new vendors to apply.

Designated sanitary control measures extend to every aspect of vending and include health requirements for everyone involved in product packaging, distribution and handling, sanitary control of the site or shop, and disposal of unsold commodities. Regulations also provide a short list of the specific items that can be distributed through outdoor vendors. Special emphasis is given to the fact that most foods should be standardized (prepacked) and prepared by workshops that fulfill the legal sanitary requirements.

The chemical and microbiological quality of all nonanimal foods is under the responsibility of the Directory of Public Health, Ministry of Health and Welfare. In the case of animal products, the Veterinary Public Health Directory, Ministry of Agriculture, is the agency in charge for safety issues. Regular inspections are conducted by health officers of the Ministry of Health and Welfare or the municipalities. If animal products are to be inspected, the veterinarians from the veterinarian authorities of the Ministry of Agriculture and the Ministry of Public Order are also involved [38].

Chemical and Microbiological Quality

No study has been conducted so far on the chemical and microbiological qualities of street foods sold in Greece. There are only limited data collected during official inspections at the places of preparation, storage, and selling. No standardized sampling methods have been used, and although the data are reliable, they are not representative of the entire production. Official inspectors assess the quality of souvlaki basically by the number of fat pieces that have been put on the skewer, and occasionally by microbiological analyses. In the area of Athens in 1996, 465 souvlaki pieces have been judged as unfit for consumption and consequently destroyed, whereas, in the first semester of 1997, 825 souvlaki and 132 cheese pie pieces did not meet the quality criteria. Total numbers of pieces inspected, however, are not available and therefore the above data cannot be used as definite [pers. commun. Police Headquarters of Athens, Department of Municipal Veterinary].

Health hazards may occur during purchase and handling of raw materials and at the various stages of street food vending. Aiming at having competitive prices, street food vendors may obtain raw materials of noncertified quality or from noncertified dealers. Storage is the next step that needs special consideration, especially when refrigeration is not available or storage facilities are easily accessible to rodents and insects. An additional problem remains the fact that most Greek street food vendors are not aware of several hygiene rules and basically prefer to act according to their personal habits and 'traditional way of doing things'. Municipalities have taken some action towards improving hygienic conditions. For instance, the usage of tongs and glass cases has been imposed to all koulouri vendors, but such measures only reach vendors who operate legally. A thorough training would be an effective mechanism in reducing risk of food contamination.

Due to the lack of scientific and official information, we turned to non-official and oral sources of information in order to discuss possible problematic aspects of the quality of Greek street foods: local press, personal communications with people who hold the inspections and 'word of mouth and popular beliefs'.

Souvlaki and Gyros

Thanks to its method of preparation, grilling, which ensures elimination of the pathogenic microorganisms, the consumption of souvlaki bears minor risks for health hazard. Furthermore, the purchased souvlaki is immediately consumed. Concerns arise when pieces of grilled meat remain unsold, are saved for future usage and not preserved properly. Consumers, however, can be warned for spoiled food by unacceptable organoleptic characteristics, such as off-flavors, texture and color. Very few cases of food intoxication due to souvlaki consumption have been reported in Greece [pers. commun., Mr. Theophanis Matralis, Veterinarian Officer].

Contrary to the souvlaki, the consumption of gyros seems to involve significant health risks for the general public. Contributing reasons for potential hazards are the difficulty in assessing organoleptically the fat content of the product or the presence of inappropriate animal tissues or parts, and the extensive use of spices and herbs that can 'mask' the unsuitability of the food. Additionally, low-scale gyros vendors habitually conserve unsold gyros at ambient temperature for several hours and use it for consumption the next day. In conclusion, four factors need to be controlled regarding the safety of pita sandwiches available: (1) type of animal tissue used; (2) microbiological quality; (3) fat content of the final product, and (4) preservation methods. The chemical quality of the oil used for the pita preparation, depending on the type of oil and the extent of reusage, is another issue which has never been addressed.

Cheese Pies

Most of the investigations on quality of cheese pies refer to adulteration problems. According to the Food and Drink Index, cheese pies are always made with *feta* cheese. The Greek *feta* is a soft brined cheese made of sheep and/or goat milk [65]. Official inspections, however, in cheese pies have recorded many other types of cheese or cheese substitutes that are less expensive and have an inferior quality. Microbiological problems can arise when cheese pies are not consumed within a few hours and are stored at ambient temperature, especially during the summer. Though data are lacking, one can speculate that cheese pies and other types of pies can be carriers of *Salmonella*, a potent food contaminant.

When discussing the microbiological quality, food handling plays an important role especially when street foods are produced by small businesses with a predominant human involvement. Human microflora reflect the environment and the habits of people who are in contact more or less with the food at all stages of its production. Potential human sources of microorganisms are the nasal cavities, mouth, and skin of food handlers.

Nuts, Seeds and Raisins

Another category of foods sold by street vendors, namely nuts and seeds, also involves potential health risk for the consumer. Peanuts, the type of nuts sold in the largest quantities, are known to be semiperishable foods. They can be kept for a relatively long time under optimum conditions, but become easily unsuitable for human consumption when stored inappropriately, due primarily to presence of molds, as well as insects, to discoloration, absorption of foreign flavors, staleness or rancidity [66]. Certain species and strains of molds that preferentially grow on peanuts produce toxins, harmful to animals and humans, known as aflatoxins. Aflatoxins are produced by certain strains of *Aspergillus flavus, Aspergilus parasiticus* and other species. Moisture and temperature are the two most important factors determining aflatoxin formation and there is a close relationship between extent of damaged kernels and aflatoxin presence [66, 67]. Once again, no data exist on prevalence of contaminated peanuts sold by street food vendors in Greece. The common practice of nut vendors to have an electric lamp on above their stalls, besides keeping their products warm, may also have a protective effect by reducing moisture content and thus aflatoxin formation.

Finally, because most of the street foods are sold outdoors with minimal precautions, they are exposed to both air and dust. This way street foods may be loaded with microcompounds potentially toxic to human health. Although no research has been conducted on this aspect of food contamination, it is highly probable for these foods to be polluted by automobile fumes and suspended particles from the road or the metro ventilation. Lead contained in vehicle exhaust gases is an issue of particular concern. It has been speculated that the amount of lead in the air, in most cases, is not sufficient to affect food displayed in open air, however, no reliable data exist and this issue deserves investigation [68]. Other possible sources of contamination include the asbestos coming from brake filings and tiny rubber pieces from tires.

Concluding Remarks

Street food vending in Greece plays a significant role in preserving a wide array of cultural traits including traditional professions, a characteristic urban infrastructure, and consumption of food items that have their roots deep in the history of the region. Street foods contribute to the vitality and local color of urban Greek centers. As a proof of that every tourist visiting this country has definitely tasted the popular Greek souvlaki, not eaten in a luxurious, comfortable restaurant, but bought from a traditional shop by the street and eaten in the street. Moreover, the Greek gyros, thanks to the business activities of the Greek immigrants, has made its way into the fast-food repertoire of most European and American cities.

The street food sector, being itself a mass feeding phenomenon, serves as the counterbalance of an expanding fast food industry. As concluded by a recent market research, the nature of the traditional mini-shops that have been selling pita sandwiches and souvlaki over the past 50 years will be carried over to the future decades unchanged [43]. The pita sandwich, in its most traditional form, will continue to supplement the Greek diet and hold its role as a staple food in modern urban Greek cities.

References

1   EKKE (Hellenic Center for Social Studies): Health and Greek Society: Descriptive Survey in a National Sample. Athens, 1988, pp 165–182.
2   Matalas A, Franti CE, Grivetti LE: Comparative study of diets and disease prevalence in Greek Chians. I. The rural and urban residents of Chios. J Food Ecol Nutr, in press.
3   Braudel F: The Structures of Everyday Life: The Wheels of Commerce. Berkeley, University of California Press, 1984, vol I, pp 79, 114–124.
4   Cheshire PC, Hay DG: Urban Problems in Western Europe. London, Unwin Hyman, 1989, pp 100–166.
5   Kostarellou E: We ate 65 billions 'fast'. Eleutherotypia, Issue of August 1995, p 43.

6   Holland B, Welch AA, Unwin ID, Buss DH, Paul AA, Southgate DAT: McCance & Widdowson's The Composition of Foods. Cambridge, Royal Society of Chemistry and MAFF, 1993.

7   Greenfield H, Lerogiannis V, Makinson J, Wills RBH: Composition of Australian foods. 19. Greek foods. Food Technol Austr 1983;35:84–86.

8   Simopoulos AP, Salem N Jr: Purslane: A terrestrial source of omega-3 fatty acids. N Engl J Med 1986;315:833.

9   Flacieliere R: The Public and Private Life of Ancient Greeks. Athens, Papademas, 1990.

10 Kalogeropoulou A: Athens in Pericle's Times. The History of the Greek Nation. Athens, Ekdotiki Athenon, 1972, vol III, p 102.

11 Durant W: Everyday Life of the Greeks. Athens, Biblos, 1954, p 307.

12 Mosse C: The End of the Athenian Republic (translation in Greek). Athens, Papazisis, 1978, pp 115–119.

13 Sarri M: The foods of ancient Greeks and their position in the financial, social and religious system of classical Greece. Archeologia 1988;28:71–74.

14 Kolobova KM, Ozereckaja EL: Everyday Life in Ancient Greece. Athens, Papademas, 1993, pp 59–60.

15 Aristophanes Acharnis: 939, 1188,1224.

16 Floros AT: Modern Greek Etymological and Interpretive Lexicon. Athens, Synora, 1980.

17 Karapli K: The wheat, the bread and the Byzantine army. Proc Symp Our bread, from wheat to bread, Pilio, ETBA, 1992.

18 Stamatakos I: Ancient Greek Language Dictionary. Athens, Bibliprometheftiki, 1990.

19 Motsias C: What ancient Greeks ate. Athens, Cactus, 1982, pp 26–28.

20 Braudel F: The Mediterranean. New York, Harper & Row, 1972.

21 Koukoules F: The Culture of the Byzantines. Athens, Collection de l'Institut Français, 1948, vol B, pp 239–242.

22 Konstantinidou M: Byzantine Streets – Traditional Cities. Athens, Selas, 1996, pp 37–40.

23 Bozi S: Cookery of the Poli. Athens, Asterismos, 1994, pp 20–24, 51, 58–63, 122–123.

24 Rice TT: The Civil and Private Life of Byzantines. Athens, Papadima, 1988.

25 Kathemereni, Issue of February 5, 1995.

26 Matalas A, Grivetti LE: The diet of nineteenth-century Greek sailors: An analysis of the log of Konstantinos. Food Foodways 1994;5:353–389.

27 Kathemerini, Smyrna. Supplement in the issue of September 14, 1997.

28 Micheli L: Erato's Notebook: The Cookery of Smyrna (1867–1919). Athens, Galatia, 1994.

29 Kairophillas Y: Athens and the Athenians. Athens, Philippotis, 1982, vol II.

30 Enepekidis PK: Confectionery in the years of Othon (presentation of a 19th century manuscript by Fredrik Unger, Royal Cook). Kathemereni, Issue of June 29.

31 Micheli L: Athens in Minor Tones. Athens, Dromena, 1987, p 122.

32 Patelis YD: Greek Professions of the Past. Athens, Paradosi, 1978, pp 90–91, 116–118.

33 Lambiki D: What Can Be Seen in Athens. Athens, Vassiliou Y Editions, 1930, pp 119–125.

34 Lozos A: Economic History of Athens. Athens, Chamber of Commerce, 1984, p 163.

35 Skaltsa MC: Social life and public sites of social gatherings in 19th century Athens. Thesis Diss, University of Thessaloniki, 1983.

36 Micheli L: Athens of the Anonymouses. Athens, Galatia, 1994, pp 42–43.

37 Flaubert G: The Voyage to Greece (December 1850–February 1851). Athens, Olkos, 1991, pp 53.

38 GMHW (Greek Ministry of Health and Welfare): On Sanitary Screening of Shops Selling Foods and Beverages, article 49. Athens, National Printing Office, 1984.

39 Tinker I: The case for legalizing street foods. Ceres 1987;20:26–31.

40 Trager J: The Food Book. New York, Flare Books, 1972, pp 25–27.

41 Fieldhouse P: Food and Nutrition: Customs and Culture. London, Chapman & Hall, 1995.

42 FAO (Food and Agriculture Organization): Food Composition Tables for the Near East. Food and Nutrition Papers, No 26. Rome, FAO, 1982.

43 ICAP: Survey on Fast Food Chains. Athens, 1997.

44 Foxall L, Forbes MR: Σιτομετρεία: The role of grain as a staple food in classical antiquity. Chiron 1982;12:41–90.

45 Trichopoulou A, Vassilakou T: Food Availability in Greece per Capita 1981–1982 and 1987–1988. Athens, National Nutrition Center Nation School of Public Health and Greek Society of Nutrition and Foods, 1995.

46 Schutz HG, Rucker MH, Russell GF: Food and food use classification systems. Food Technol 1975; 29:50–64.

47 Kopulos S, Jones PD: Adventures on Greek Cookery. New York, World Publishing, 1966, pp 1–19.

48 Anonymous: The Dinner Philosopher. Athens, Ikaros, 1991, pp 21–26.

49 Efimeris Kyverniseos 1995;145:2323, article 1.

50 Tinker I, Cohen M: Street foods as a source of income for women. Ekistics 1985;310:83–89.

51 FAO (Food and Agriculture Organization): Women in food production, food handling and nutrition, with special emphasis on Africa: A report of the protein-calorie advisory group of the United Nations system. Rome, FAO, 1979, pp 118–122.

52 FAO (Food and Agriculture Organization): Street Foods. Food, Nutrition and Agriculture Series, No 17/18. Rome, FAO, 1996.

53 ESYE (National Statistical Office of Greece): Household Budget Survey 1993–1994. Official Bulletin, 1997.

54 Jelliffe DB: Parallel food classifications in developing and industrialized countries. Am J Clin Nutr 1967;20:279–281.

55 Solomons NW, Gross R: Urban nutrition in developing countries. Nutr Rev 1995;53:90–95.

56 Lennernäs M, Fjellström C, Becker W, Giachetti I, Schmitt A, Remaut de Winter AM, Kearney M: Influences on food choice perceived to be important by nationally-representative samples of adults in the European Union. Eur J Clin Nutr 1997;51(suppl 2):S8–S15.

57 Winamo FG, Allain A: Street foods in developing countries: Lessons from Asia. Food Nutr Agric/FAO 1991;1:11–18.

58 WHO (World Health Organization): Essential Safety Requirements for Street-Vended Foods. Geneva, WHO, 1996.

59 Dubisch J (ed): Culture enters through the kitchen: Women, food and social boundaries in rural Greece; in Dubisch C (ed): Gender and Power in Rural Greece. Princeton, Princeton University Press, 1986, pp 203–205.

60 Paige DM (ed): Nutritional analyses of fast-foods; in Paige DM (ed): Clinical Nutrition. St. Louis, Mosby, 1988.

61 Jansen A, Menotti A, Nedeljkovic S, Pekkarinen M, Simic BS, Toshima H: Food consumption patterns in the 1960s in seven countries. Am J Clin Nutr 1989;49:889–894.

62 Sabate J, Fraser GE, Burke K, Knutsen SF, Bennett H, Lindsted KD: Effects of walnuts on serum lipid levels and blood pressure in normal men. N Engl J Med 1993;328:603–607.

63 Dreher ML, Maher CV, Kearney P: The traditional and emerging role of nuts in healthful diets. Nutr Rev 1996;54:241–245.

64 Tee ES: Carotenoids and retinoids in human nutrition. Crit Rev Food Sci Nutr 1992;31:103–163.

65 USDA (US Department of Agriculture): Cheese Varieties and Description. Agricultural Handbook No 54, Agricultural Eastern Utilization Research and Development Division, Agricultural Research Service. Washington, 1953, p 44.

66 Woodroof JG: Peanuts: Production Processing Products. Westport, AVI Publishing, 1966, pp 85–111.

67 Jay MJ: Modern Food Microbiology. New York, Chapman & Hall, 1996, pp 595–600.

68 Abdussalam M, Käferstein FK: Safety of street foods. World Health Forum 1993;14:191–194.

Antonia-Leda Matalas, Department of Nutrition and Dietetics, Harokopio University, El. Venizelou 70, GR–17671 Athens (Greece)

Simopoulos AP, Bhat RV (eds): Street Foods.
World Rev Nutr Diet. Basel, Karger, 2000, vol 86, pp 25–44

....

Street Foods in America – A True Melting Pot

Denise S. Taylor, Valerie K. Fishell, Jessica L. Derstine,
Rebecca L. Hargrove, Natalie R. Patterson, Kristin W. Moriarty,
Beverly A. Battista, Hope E. Ratcliffe, Amy E. Binkoski,
Penny M. Kris-Etherton

Graduate Program in Nutrition, The Pennsylvania State University, University Park, Pa., USA

Many different foods from all of the food groups are available from street food vendors. Moreover, there is a wide variety of ethnic foods sold by street vendors representing cuisines that reflect the ethnic diversity of the local population and customs. Because of the vast array of food choices available and relatively unknown consumption patterns, there is little information about the contribution of these foods to the diet of Americans. Thus, this paper will provide an overview of the foods available and the health, safety and regulatory issues associated with consumption of street foods. Because of limited information about street foods in the American diet, it is obvious that we have much to learn about how these foods impact on the American diet and, in turn, the health status of the population. It is not unreasonable to speculate that these foods may play a more prominent role in the US diet in the future because of changing lifestyles. Consequently, more information is needed about availability, consumption practices, impact on energy and nutrient intake, and the safety of street foods. In this paper, we discuss these important issues and identify issues that the nutrition community needs to address about street foods.

Historical Perspective of Street Food Vending

Street vendors, throughout history, have endured a love-hate relationship with the cities in which they work. For example, in 1930 one supporter of street vendors declared, 'The pushcart marketers are as characteristic a part of the New York pageant as the skyscrapers' [1], yet others blamed pushcarts for contributing to traffic congestion, stealing business from local stores, and stigmatizing neighborhoods, thereby reducing real estate values [2]. New York City serves as an excellent historical model for this love-hate relationship, since it has developed regulations to control yet maintain street vending, and street vendors have adapted to continue their unique way of selling goods.

Street vendors have been battling city magistrates as far back as the 17th century to maintain a place on the streets and make a living for themselves and their families. In 1691, a New York City ordinance forbade street vendors, otherwise known as 'hucksters', from selling goods until after public markets had been open for 2 h. By 1707, street food vendors were completely banned from the streets of New York City [3]. Many of the proposals to ban street vendors came about to prevent congestion on the streets and to allow the roadways to serve only as traffic throughways. In addition, retail stores and restaurants complained about the presence of street vendors because they stole business by parking in front of stores and restaurants. As such, one regulation forbade vendors from occupying the same spot for more than 15 min. Despite these strict laws, street vendors still flourished as police and property owners either extorted money from vendors or were paid off to ignore regulations, allowing street vendors to conduct 'business as usual' [4].

Between 1827 and 1846 retail stores, department stores, and specialty shops opened, and middle- and upper-class consumers moved inside to do their shopping [5]. The street vendor market became a business that the lower class maintained, both as vendors and consumers. A high percentage of these vendors were foreign, specifically European immigrants from Ireland, Italy and Greece as well as Jewish immigrants from Russia, Poland and Romania. Since most of the immigrants had no marketable skills and did not know English, the neighborhood-based pushcart markets gave recent immigrants a familiar cultural and linguistic setting in which to earn a living. In the 1890s, the peddling of goods, including food, was the second largest occupation among the Jewish community [6]. In 1925, 32 and 63% of the fruit and vegetable peddlers were Italian and Jewish, respectively [7]. Many continued in the trade for ten or more years, spending long hours in adverse conditions for very little compensation in hopes of one day owning a business in a fixed location.

Street vending rose to prominence in New York City in the 1880s and then was almost completely abolished during the 1930s. Throughout this period many economic and social changes took place that had a tremendous impact on the view of street vendors' place in society. During the period from 1880 to 1901, street vendors chose to ignore the regulation that restricted the amount of time they could spend in one place and started selling continuously from a single location. Several vendors took up adjacent positions along a street and informal markets were formed [8]. This system soon spread throughout New York City. In 1913, the city designated specific areas such as the approaches to Manhattan, Williamsburg and Queensboro bridges as street-vending areas [4]. This was a further affempt to control the street vendors. Following World War I, New York City legalized and expanded the street-vending markets in an attempt to confine them to designated streets. Between 1920 and 1924, twenty-three street markets were in operation and by the early 1930s, this number had jumped to 60 [2]. However, the attitude toward street vendors turned in the late 1930s when the LaGuardia administration abolished nearly all of the existing street markets and built several enclosed market buildings in an attempt to 'tidy up the streets' [9] in time for the World's Fair. By the end of 1939, only 17 markets remained and the number of vendor licenses declined from 7,000 to just over 1,000 [2]. Only a small part of the once thriving vendors' markets survived into the 1940s. In 1946, ten vendor markets still operated and by 1964 this number had dropped to six [10]. Now, even in the 1990s, vendors in New York City and other US cities face opposition from government officials (see 'Regulatory issues' section).

Despite opposition, street vending has survived and changed throughout its history. There has been a transition from vendors selling foods from horse-drawn and wheelbarrow wagons to the practices seen today of using pushcarts or trucks with panels that open on the side to set up business. In the 1920s and 1930s, street food vendors sold farm products, most commonly fruits and vegetables, from horse-drawn wagons. Sometimes, however, less typical food items such as cottage cheese were sold. Ice cream wagons that vended through neighborhoods also became quite popular, with ice cream packed in a bucket of ice and distributed from the wagon. With the development of refrigeration, the ice cream truck became more modernized and ice cream was served from within the truck where it was kept cold. Other accounts of neighborhood street food vendors include a butcher who traveled through the streets in a wagon selling meat to families. Milk was also delivered in this fashion. Of course, these foods were not ready-prepared meals as one might find on the city streets of America today; however, this neighborhood delivery system evolved into the development of ready-made foods to be consumed at the point of purchase.

Interestingly, several restaurant chains began as single, street food stands. Once vendors outgrew their facilities, they were forced to move to buildings and eventually became national franchises. For example, McDonald's was a single hamburger stand in Pasadena, Calif. in 1940 and became the restaurant in 1948 [11]. Orange Julius, which was originally an orange juice stand opened by Julius Freed in Los Angeles in 1925, later developed into a franchise featuring a unique, orange frothy drink. The franchise has flourished, spreading throughout the US and into Canada. Now run under the Dairy Queen franchise, Orange Julius cafes can be found in shopping malls throughout North America [11]. Stuckey's also started out as a roadside stand that sold pecans. William Sylvester Stuckey ran the stand, but when his wife started making fudge and candies to sell with the pecans, they soon grew out of their stand and opened the retail candy store known today as Stuckey's [11].

The business of street food vending has changed significantly over time, especially with respect to regulations on street food vendors, as well as the way by which street vendors sell their foods. With the exception of jingling ice cream trucks that ride through neighborhoods on summer evenings, street food vending presently entails consumers visiting mobile food carts on city streets to consume food at the point of purchase. The carts and trucks which street food vendors use are relatively standard, as are the regulations that ensure safety and quality of food sold on the street. Some traditional foods that were sold on the streets during the beginning of this century, such as hamburgers, nuts and fresh fruits, are still favorite street foods. In addition to traditional street foods, however, many more ethnic selections and entire meals are available for purchase on the street today.

Types of Foods Sold on the Street

Just as America is the melting pot for all people, cultures and heritages, so too are the foods found on America's city streets. In large metropolitan areas throughout the US one can find an array of foods ranging from the ever-popular American soft pretzels and hot dogs to Italian sausage sandwiches, Mexican burritos, Middle Eastern falafels, and Chinese egg rolls (table 1). This cornucopia of cultures and food selections reflects the diversity of tastes and lifestyles of each city.

Four of the predominant cultural selections reflecting an internationalization of food in America include Italian, Mexican, Middle Eastern and Chinese foods. However, many other cultural foods are offered on the streets, such as Navajo fry bread, German bratwursts, Greek gyro and souvlaki, Indian samosas, Japanese yakitori, Caribbean roti and patties, and Argentine empanadas.

One of the primary cultural selections, Italian food, includes favorites such as stromboli, Italian sausage and meatball sandwiches, hoagies, and various pasta dishes. Mexican street food also has become a favorite for many Americans, with hot items such as burritos, tacos, chili, Spanish rice and nachos packed to eat on the street. For many of the typically meat-

Table 1. Typical foods found on city streets

American	*Italian*
Bagel	Calzone
Baked potato	Italian hoagie (Sub)
Cheeseburger	Meatball sandwich
Cheesecake	Pasta
Cheese steak	Sausage sandwich
Chicken breast	Stromboli
Corn-on-the-cob	
French fries	*Mexican*
Fried shrimp	Burrito
Hamburger	Chili
Hoagie (Sub)	Nachos
Hot dog	Spanish rice
Ice cream	Taco
Muffin	
Nuts	*Middle Eastern*
Pizza	Baba ghannouj
Slurpie/Smoothie	Falafel
Soft pretzel	Fried eggplant
Soup	Hummus
Sticky bun	
Wings	*Other*
	Argentine empanada
Chinese	Caribbean roti and patty
Bamboo-wrapped rice	German bratwurst
Beef tripe	Greek gyro
Crab sticks	Spanish churro
Egg drop soup	Indian samosa
Egg roll	Japanese yakitori
Fried rice	Philippine lumpia
Gyoza	Cappuccino and espresso
Lo mein	Doughnuts and pastries
Tempura	Fresh fruit
Wonton soup	

based selections such as chili, tacos and burritos, vendors may offer beef, chicken and vegetarian bean varieties in order to appeal to many tastes and preferences.

Middle Eastern selections also appeal to those seeking a change from the typical, American fast-food hamburgers and hot dogs. The most popular Middle Eastern street food, falafel, is a deep-fried patty consisting of chick peas and tahini (a sesame seed paste), that is often tucked inside a pita pocket with chopped cucumbers, cabbage and tomatoes. Other popular selections include cubed, skinless, fried eggplant and hummus.

In Chinese-American neighborhoods throughout the US, and particularly in Manhattan's Chinatown, vendors prepare traditional Chinese dishes on hot griddles and steam tables [12]. Along with the popular egg rolls and wonton soup, one also may find lo mein, beef tripe, gyoza (vegetable dumplings), fried rice and tempura (batter-fried vegetable patties). Other unusual choices may include marble-sized fish balls atop large rice noodles or warm sweet rice wrapped inside bamboo leaves.

In addition to the diverse cultural foods available on the street, not to be overlooked are the common American street foods which are synonymous with the names of many cities. For example, Philadelphia owes much of its notoriety to the one-of-a-kind Philly cheese steak and popular Philly soft pretzel. For just thirty-five cents (or three for a dollar), one can indulge in a large Philly soft pretzel with mustard. Additional favorite Philadelphia street foods include sticky buns and hoagies (i.e. subs). New York City is known for its all-American hot dog stands, which abound on many street corners. Additionally, the aroma of fresh roasted peanuts allures many passers-by, while roasted chestnuts, that are sold particularly during the Christmas holiday season, appeal to busy, hungry New York shoppers.

College towns also provide a strong market for street food vendors. For example, in Ithaca, New York, home to Cornell University and Ithaca College, a favorite lunchtime stop, 'Louie's Lunch Wagon', draws crowds of students and returning alumni to purchase pizza, wings, nachos and chili dogs from the famous venda-truck. At many universities, especially those on the West Coast, street food vendors sell coffee, Danish, biscotti, bagels and muffins to students looking for a quick bite and caffeine jolt before their next class. Several college towns boast 'Burrito Buggies', where students can grab a wrapped-up meal between classes or late-night snack after the bars have closed.

In Los Angeles, pizza and ice cream vendors walk through the streets ringing bells to lure passing crowds to purchase their delicious treats. Popsicles and ice cream bars are a favorite commodity sold throughout the city to help beat the heat. Given its warm climate and large Hispanic population, Los Angeles also has unique street foods including year-round fresh oranges and mangos, as well as authentic Mexican food.

Other common American foods often sold on the street include packaged foods such as pretzels, chips, nuts and muffins as well as prepared baked, fried and grilled foods such as shishkebobs, ribs and corn-on-the-cob. One may also select from an assortment of beverages ranging from hot coffee, espresso, cappuccino, tea and cocoa to cold sodas and frozen slurpies. Street vendors may also tempt passing crowds with a myriad of desserts including cinnamon buns, ice cream, chocolate, cakes and cookies.

In addition to the many cultural and popular American street foods, some vendors offer alternatives for health-conscious consumers. As opposed to high-fat french fries, doughnuts, and candy bars found at many street carts, certain vendors offer low-fat choices such as baked potatoes, pretzels, bagels, water-ice, pasta salads and fresh fruits. In New York City, for example, many tourists and businesspersons flock to the 'Potato King' for a quick lunch. While a large baked potato can provide a healthy snack or meal at about 200 calories, the toppings can make or break the potato. The 'Potato King' offers a few low-fat choices such as vegetables and chives, but the more popular choices are high-fat toppings such as cheese, sour cream, bacon, butter and chili. Similarly, a plain bagel can serve as a low-fat snack, but if loaded with regular cream cheese, its nutrient profile begins to resemble a high-fat muffin or doughnut. On the other hand, fresh fruit carts offer convenient, almost always guaranteed low-fat, vitamin-packed snacks, that burst with flavor when in season.

No longer does one have to go to a sports stadium to enjoy the aroma of fresh roasted peanuts and hot dogs, nor to a tucked-away ethnic restaurant or international market to taste ethnic foods such as Middle-Eastern falafels or Argentine empenadas, nor even to the supermarket for fresh fruits. These foods, along with a variety of other popular 'street treats' [13], are available from street food vendors in most major American cities. Whether a city native, weekday commuter, or visitor, the variety and accessibility of street foods provide something for everyone.

Nutritional Analysis of Selected Street Foods

Due to the wide range of street-vended foods available in US cities, it is difficult to generally assess their nutritional value. Obviously, the food choices consumers make largely determine the nutritional value of street foods. Data from USDA's 1995 Continuing Survey of Food Intakes by Individuals (CSFII) does indicate, however, that foods eaten away from home tend to be higher in fat, saturated fat, cholesterol and sodium, and lower in fiber and calcium than foods eaten at home [14]. For example, this survey indicated that home foods averaged 34.7 g of fat and 12 g of saturated fat per 1,000 calories as compared to 41.8 g of fat and 14.3 g of saturated fat for away-from-home foods.

Although the contribution of street-vended foods to the consumption of away-from-home foods is unclear, many street foods are high in fat and saturated fat. Table 2 summarizes the nutritional value of some foods commonly

Table 2. Nutritional profile of selected street foods[1]

Food item	Energy kcal	Total fat % energy	SFA % energy	MUFA % energy	PUFA % energy	Linoleic acid $C_{18:2}$ g	Linolenic acid $C_{18:3}$ g
American							
Bagel (1, 4″ diameter)	245	5	0.7	0.4	2	0.59	0.03
Baked potato, plain (1 large)	220	0.8	–	–	–	–	
Baked potato with cheese sauce (1)	474	55	20	20	11	–	–
Baked potato with sour cream and chives (1)	393	51	23	18	8	–	–
Cheese pizza (1 slice)	140	21	10	6	3	0.44	0.06
Chestnuts (1 oz)	68	4	0.7	2	1	0.08	0.01
Hot dog (1 sandwich)	242	54	19	25	6	1.28	0.42
Peanuts, dry-roasted (1 oz)	166	76	11	38	24	4.45	0.001
Soft pretzel (1)	190	8	3	4	0.7	–	–
Submarine sandwich	456	37	13	16	5	–	–
Chinese							
Chow mein noodles (1 cup)	237	53	7	13	30	6.91	0.89
Egg roll (1)	114	49	12	21	12	–	–
Fried rice (1 serving)	197	18	5	6	5	0.99	0.03
Italian							
Italian sausage, pork (1 link)	216	72	25	33	9	1.90	0.30
Stromboli (1)	241	37	17	10	6	0.84	0.11
Mexican							
Bean and cheese burrito (2)	378	28	16	6	4	1.58	0.21
Beef burrito (2)	524	36	18	13	1.5	0.77	0.09
Chili (1 cup)	256	29	12	12	2	0.30	0.23
Nachos with cheese (6–8)	346	49	20	21	6	2.04	0.20
Taco (1 small)	369	50	28	16	2	0.88	0.08
Middle Eastern							
Falafel (1 patty)	57	48	6	27	11	0.08	0.02
Hummus (1 T)	23	53	–	–	–	–	–
Other							
Navajo fry bread (1, 5″ diameter)	296	26	5	8	11	3.35	0.21
Bratwurst, pork (1 link)	256	77	28	36	8	2.11	0.22

[1] USDA nutrient database values were used for all foods except for soft pretzel, stromboli, egg roll and fried rice, for which Nutritionist IV was used.

sold by street vendors. These analyses were performed using the online USDA nutrient database and Nutritionist IV (Version 4.1, Copyright 1995, First Databank Division, San Bruno, Calif., USA). Fast foods items were used where applicable. Clearly, the nutrient content of street foods will vary with the use of different ingredients and preparation techniques, but these analyses provide an estimate of potential fat intake from typical street foods. Many of the foods listed, such as hot dogs, egg rolls, stromboli and nachos, have greater than 30% of calories from fat and are high in saturated fat as well.

Despite the prevalence of high-fat street foods, other food choices are available to the health-conscious consumer. According to table 2, a bagel, plain baked potato, slice of cheese pizza, ounce of chestnuts, soft pretzel, navajo fry bread, and even a serving of fried rice each contribute less than 30% of calories from fat and 10% or less from saturated fat. For instance, a soft pretzel contains approximately 190 calories and only 1.7 g of fat and 0.6 g of saturated fat. A dab of mustard would only add a few calories and no fat. However, condiments can make a huge difference in the nutritional quality of street foods. For example, a baked potato with cheese sauce provides 474 calories and 55% of calories from fat as compared to a plain baked potato with 220 calories and 0.8% calories from fat. Similarly, cheese pizza is a healthy street food choice at 140 calories, 3.3 g of fat, and 1.6 g of saturated fat. However, if pepperoni or sausage is added, the nutritional profile of the piece of pizza reflects a higher calorie, higher fat choice. Moreover, one slice of cheese pizza looks nutritionally appealing, but if two or three pieces are eaten – which is more realistic of the typical American consumer – calories, total fat and saturated fat obviously double or triple.

Recently there has been considerable interest in the contribution of monounsaturated and polyunsaturated fat to the American diet. Roasted peanuts are an excellent source of these types of fat, contributing 38% of calories as monounsaturated fat and 24% of calories as polyunsaturated fat per 1-ounce serving. Although food preparation techniques vary among vendors, the main sources of the polyunsaturated omega-3 (n–3) and omega-6 (n–6) fatty acids from street foods are those foods prepared with vegetable oils, such as soybean oil and corn oil. As shown in table 2, chow mein noodles are an excellent source of n–3 and n–6 fatty acids, providing 0.89 g of linolenic acid and 6.91 g of linoleic acid per 1-cup serving, respectively. Tahini, a ground sesame seed paste, which is used in falafel and hummus, is also a good source of linoleic acid, providing 3.47 g per tablespoon.

Although the contribution of street foods to the American diet is not clear, such foods may be a regular component of the meals of some Americans or may simply provide them with a quick snack. For example, a businessperson in New York City may grab a bagel or muffin and coffee from a street food vendor on his or her way to work every morning. In order for consumers to make healthful food choices, nutrition education and nutrition labeling of street-vended foods is needed. Presently, nutrition information of foods sold by street food vendors is rarely available at the point of purchase. Displaying nutritional information will help consumers make more informed choices about the foods they eat away from home.

Preparation and Processing of Street Foods

By definition, 'street foods (and beverages) are prepared and/or sold by vendors in streets and other public places for immediate consumption or consumption at a later time without further processing or preparation' [15]. Thus, the extent of preparation and processing of street foods is minimal, but still is an essential part of ensuring the sale of a safe product.

The 1996 WHO Food Safety Unit Report on the essential safety requirements for street-vended foods states that proper preparation and processing techniques are essential to ensuring the safety of street-vended foods. Three critical roles of preparation and processing were identified in the report [15]:

(1) Preparation and processing should be adequate to eliminate or reduce hazards to an acceptable level.

(2) Preparation and processing should prevent growth of pathogens, production of toxic chemicals and the introduction of physical hazards.

(3) Preparation and processing should ensure that foods are not recontaminated.

Preparation and processing will also affect the nutritional quality of foods via their influence on nutrient loss. Although fat-soluble vitamins and minerals are generally fairly stable, water-soluble vitamins are easily lost in preparation, processing and storage. Vitamin C, thiamin and folate are especially susceptible to being lost or destroyed [16].

Exposure to heat, air and light, as well as cooking with water and baking soda, all contribute to nutrient losses and should be kept to a minimum. The fresher the food, the more nutrient dense it will be, which is especially true of perishable fruits and vegetables. In addition, cutting fruits and vegetables into small pieces results in increased surface area exposed to heat, oxygen and water, which results in increased nutrient loss due to leaching and oxidation. Thus, the ideal situation entails cooking fresh, whole foods at the lowest possible temperature, using the least amount of water. Consumption of food immediately or shortly thereafter also is recommended to minimize nutrient losses.

Table 3. Foodborne disease outbreaks due to bacteria as a % of outbreaks of known etiology and % of total outbreaks – US and Canada

	Total outbreaks	Total outbreaks with known etiology	Total outbreaks due to bacteria	% of outbreaks of known etiology due to bacteria	% of total outbreaks due to bacteria
USA					
1973–1987 [20]	7,458	2,841	1,869	66	25
1988–1992 [21]	2,423	1,001	796	80	33
*Canada**					
1975–1984 [22]	8,672	2,109	1,381	65	16
1985–1986 [23]	2,236	601	392	65	18

*Canadian data are reported as total outbreaks due to microbiological factors and includes outbreaks due to viral infections.

Microbial Quality of Street Foods

No studies have been conducted that characterize the microbial quality of street foods in the US and Canada, and presently no convincing evidence exists that street foods are more responsible for the transmission of foodborne infection and intoxication [17] than foods obtained elsewhere. As such, inferences have been drawn from studies examining the microbial quality of foods prepared in foodservice establishments that are similar to those sold as street foods. For example, of the 1,600 cases of food poisoning reported by physicians to the New York City Health Department during 1992 and 1993, only eight were suspected to be from street foods. Of these eight, only one case was actually proven to be food poisoning and even this case could not definitely be tied to street foods [18]. However, this does not infer that foodborne illness from street foods could not or does not occur. Risk of foodborne illness from street foods is implied if one looks at the occurrence of foodborne illness attributed to foods served in restaurants that are similar to foods sold by street vendors.

Bryan [19] reviewed foodborne disease surveillance data from the US for the years 1977 through 1984 to determine the relative importance of various foods as vehicles of foodborne disease and found that the most frequently implicated foods were beef (roast and ground beef in particular), pork (ham in particular), chicken, and Chinese and Mexican-style foods. Other foodborne disease outbreak surveillance summaries conducted in the US found results

Table 4. Foods associated with foodborne incidents in the US and Canada, by specific agents[a]

	Meat	Poultry	Chinese	Mexican	Total[b]
US 1973–1992					
B. cereus	4	4	36	5	79
C. perfringens	69	34	0	27	224
Salmonella	121	85	4	18	1,062
S. aureus	134	36	3	6	416
Canada 1975–1986					
B. cereus	11	10	66	NA[c]	152
C. perfringens	73	30	1	NA	182
Salmonella	56	193	12	NA	606
S. aureus	93	50	12	NA	353

[a] Information obtained from references 20, 21, 22 and 23.
[b] Total incidents attributed to each specific pathogen.
[c] Information for Canada not available.

similar to those of Bryan [20, 21]. Todd [22, 23] compiled summaries of surveillance information on foodborne diseases occurring in Canada between 1975 and 1986 and found results very similar to those reported in the US. As shown in table 3, bacterial infection accounts for a majority of the total outbreaks of foodborne illness in the US and Canada. Therefore, reducing the incidents of bacterial infections would greatly reduce the incidents of foodborne illness.

The pathogens most frequently associated with foodborne illness linked to foodservice establishments were *Bacillus cereus, Clostridium perfringens, Salmonella,* and *Staphylococcus aureus* [23]. Table 4 shows the foods most associated with foodborne illness incidents and the specific pathogens responsible. In both the US and Canada, Chinese food is the most likely source of foodborne illness due to *B. cereus,* while meat and poultry are likely sources of foodborne illness due to *C. perfringens* and *S. aureus.* Table 5 depicts foodborne disease outbreaks by etiology and contributing factors. The contributing factors most responsible for outbreaks include, but are not limited to: improper holding temperature, inadequate cooking, and poor personal hygiene. From this information, inferences can easily be made about the microbial quality of street foods as these or similar foods are commonly sold as street foods in the US and Canada. Many other foods, such as gyros, Chinese duck, cold salads and pizza, because of their composi-

Table 5. Foodborne disease outbreaks by etiology and contributing factors
– US 1988–1992 [21]

	Number of reported outbreaks	Factors reported[1]	Improper holding temperature	Inadequate cooking	Poor personal hygiene
B. cereus	21	16	16	4	2
C. perfringens	40	33	31	13	1
Salmonella	549	372	215	191	143
S. aureus	50	42	37	15	18
Total bacterial	796	537	329	257	183

[1] More than one factor can contribute to an outbreak.

tion and preparation practices, are also potential vehicles for foodborne illness.

A joint FAO/WHO Expert Committee on Food Safety was convened to study the potential hazards of street-vended foods [24]. The Committee concluded that the best approach to food safety for street foods was the use of the Hazard Analysis and Critical Control Point (HACCP) system to identify behaviors and practices which may be hazardous. The HACCP approach is based on understanding: (1) the factors that contribute to outbreaks of foodborne illness; (2) the problems associated with food additives and chemical contaminants, and (3) the presence of foreign objects. A hazard is defined as an unacceptable contamination of a microbial, chemical or physical nature, and/or unacceptable survival or persistence, and/or unacceptable growth or increase of microbes. Therefore, a logical step toward reducing the risk of foodborne illness from street foods would be controlling the steps involved in food preparation and sale that may contribute to the contamination, survival or growth of the microbes responsible for foodborne illness.

Bryan's group conducted hazard analysis of gyros [25], fried rice [26], roast pork [27], and Chinese duck [28] in restaurants and found that all of these foods, like many other foods sold by street vendors, have the potential to cause serious problems unless handled properly. In addition, hazard analysis of street foods in countries other than the US and Canada [29–35] indicates that while the foods are different from country to country, the hazards identified in the preparation and sale of the cooked foods were very similar. The major hazards for cooked foods were identified as: (1) handling cooked foods with bare hands; (2) preparing cooked foods on surfaces previously used for raw foods without cleaning between uses; (3) holding foods that should be refrigerated or held hot at outdoor or indoor ambient temperatures for many hours, and (4) insufficiently reheating foods. Street food vendors are often poor, uneducated and may lack the appreciation of safe food handling. If communities are to enjoy the benefits of street-vended foods, food safety activities must concentrate on teaching those who handle, prepare, process and store street foods about specific hazards and means by which control can be applied at each critical control point. While health department regulations on licensed street food vendors address these issues, the plethora of unlicensed vendors on the street may compromise the safety and quality of street foods.

Regulatory Issues Surrounding Street Food Vending

Health department regulations, either at the state, county or city level of government, clearly define different types of mobile food establishments and describe sanitary procedures that must be employed with each type of food cart. The application for and issuance of licenses/permits for street food vendors, including the inspection of their carts, fall under health department (or similar agency) regulations. Beyond the basic infrastructure of health department regulations on street foods, which generally target food safety and quality, it is important to consider other regulations that have resulted from the rapid growth of the street food business. In particular, local laws and specific Internal Revenue Service (IRS) initiatives to enforce proper tax payment provide examples of the recent crackdown on street food vendors.

Since regulations vary among the states and because New York City probably houses more street food vendors than any other US city, New York City Health Department regulations will be discussed as an example. In the state of New York, street food vendors must obtain a valid permit from the health department for lawful operation of mobile food carts. Depending on the population of the location where the food is to be vended, the permit-issuing official may be the city or county health commissioner or the state regional health director [36]. Since New York City's population is well above 50,000, the New York City Department of Health has jurisdiction over street food vendors in the city. Before food can be lawfully vended on the streets, the prospective vendor must pay a fee to the health department and file an application, which includes a list of all foods that will be served. On the vending application, the potential vendor must also supply the name of the approved commissary or restaurant where the vendor will obtain his or her food. Once the application has been approved and the mobile food service establishment has been inspected, a permit is issued for 1 year and must be prominently displayed on the vendor's mobile food cart. The permit-issuing official may inspect mobile food carts at any time, with failure to meet health department regulations as grounds for suspension or revoking of a vendor's permit. Further, if a street food vendor is found operating a mobile food cart without a permit from the health department, they can be ordered to immediately cease all food services.

Currently, the number of people seeking street food vending permits in New York City exceeds the number of permits available [37]. As a result, a lottery system is in place to determine who gets a permit and who does not. Realistically, many street food vendors bypass this system altogether and sell their food illegally (i.e. without a permit) on the street, remaining transient to avoid prosecution.

In addition to health department regulations, various local laws have been adopted to deal with the overcrowding of streets and sidewalks by food vendors. In the 1980s in Washington D.C., a policy was enforced to remove two of every three vendors from the streets. The cost for licenses increased, the number handed out declined, and stricter regulations were enforced on the foods that could be sold on the street. In 1996, also in Washington D.C., a law was passed by the County Council which prohibits the Office of Business and Regulatory Affairs from issuing any new street food vending licenses [38]. Furthermore, Washington D.C. street food vendors are prohibited from selling food within 100 yards of an intersection [38]. In Chicago, a 1991 proposed ordinance restricted mobile food vendors from operating within 200 feet of a restaurant and limited them to two hours of operation in any spot [39]. This ordinance would eliminate vendors almost entirely from the Chicago Loop area because of the high concentration of restaurants.

New York City may have one of the most restrictive local laws on street food vendors. Regulation 11, which was passed in 1983, barred vendors from over 100 streets in midtown Manhattan. The law, which was enacted to prevent the congestion of food vendors in crowded New York streets, was rarely enforced because New Yorkers, in particular, enjoy street food [40]. More recently, however, New York City is targeting street food vendors by pressing the police to enforce this 15-year-old law [41].

Local authorities are not alone in their crack down on street food vendors –the IRS is taking a closer look at tax payments made by street food vendors. An IRS-launched program entitled Compliance 2000 earmarks street food vendors, especially the new wave of coffee cart vendors on the west coast, as individuals who may be avoiding or underpaying taxes. The transient nature of street food vending and the large number of vendors working illegally contribute to the frustration the IRS faces when trying to track down these individuals. Many cities, such as New York and Los Angeles, keep track of street food vendors by requiring them to obtain a tax identification card or retail sales business tax registration certificate to legally sell their foods on the street. This card or certificate is required in addition to a license or permit and is used in accordance with the payment of business tax.

Along with the variety of ethnic, convenient and inexpensive food offered by street food vendors comes the problems of congestion on the streets and sidewalks, business being taken away from restaurants, and illegal vendor activities, such as selling food without a permit and avoiding/underpaying taxes. Health department regulations, local laws, and IRS initiatives are in place to address some of these important issues, but the burdens of monitoring street food vending are still challenging. Better enforcement of existing regulations and development of effective, new regulations on street food vendors are clearly needed; however, the unique flavor and flair of city street foods must not be compromised.

Profile of Street Food Vendors and Consumers

In urban communities, the sale of street foods is an important source of income for vendors. Numerous vendors have no other skills to enter the job market and use their income to support their family in the United States and abroad. Street food vendors represent a variety of ethnic groups and include immigrants from countries such as India, Lebanon, Korea, Pakistan, Vietnam and Mexico. Many immigrant vendors view peddling as a temporary job and the first step into the job market in America. They may avoid the legal aspects of street food vending (e.g. green cards, permits/licenses and tax forms) by working in heavy vending areas, such as New York City, San Francisco, Philadelphia and Washington D.C. [37]. Due to the massive number of vendors in these areas, it is more difficult for officials to regulate food vendors, thus making it easier for illegal vendors to work the streets.

Women play a relatively minor role in the vending of street foods in America, unlike their prominent role in developing countries [42]. There are minimal accounts of women selling foods on the streets; however, women were often behind the scenes, baking goods and candies to be sold on the streets by their husbands. In the 1980s in Washington, D.C., only 1 in 5 street vendors was female. 40% were Caucasian, while the other 60% were either African American, Latino or Asian [44].

In a recent study on Manhattan's 14th Street vendor's market [37], 1 of 8 licensed hot-food vendors was female and almost all fruit-cart vendors were men, whereas at least three out of ten unlicensed cold-food vendors were women. Unlicensed cold-food vendors tended to be of lower socioeconomic status than other vendors on 14th Street and they prepared various food items at home. These findings are probably typical of most North American cities, where a higher proportion of the unlicensed food vendors are immigrant women, who sell food prepared in their homes to support their families who may or may not be in the country [38].

Aside from fruit carts, most vendors operate during lunch and dinner hours, roughly 10:30 a.m. through 6:00 p.m., and work 6 days a week. Fruit cart vendors, on the other hand, are often seen during weekday morning hours, trying to attract people on their way to work. Fruit cart vendors are scarce during the winter months in many northern metropolitan cities due to limited availability of seasonable fruits and the inability to hold fruit at winter temperatures, which often fall below the freezing point.

Street foods provide ready-to-eat and fairly inexpensive snacks and meals for a wide variety of people. People who work in downtown areas, as well as students and shoppers, are regular consumers of street foods. For these people, returning home for a meal may not be possible due to lack of time and/or congested roads and overcrowded public transportation systems. Convenient street foods provide a welcomed alternative to cooking, particularly for women who are under increased time constraints while striving to balance home and work. In addition, single men are likely consumers of street foods because they may be less inclined to cook for themselves. Street foods may also be essential in the food supply of low-income persons, particularly those who do not have a place in which to prepare food. Many tourists appreciate the culturally unique foods that are sold on the street. Lastly, even health-conscious consumers purchase street foods as vendors accommodate their needs by providing low-fat foods and a variety of vegetarian items.

As people spend more time working away from their homes, they tend to eat out more often. According to the Restaurant Industry Report of 1993 [45], the average American family spent 36% of its food budget on meals and snacks outside the home, an increase from 25% in 1950. Interestingly, the typical person eats 3.5 meals per week away from home [45], and fast foods account for 43% of all meals eaten away from home [14]. Unfortunately, no specific category presently exists to quantify the consumption of street foods.

Clearly, difficulties lie not only in identifying who actually buys and sells street foods, but also to what extent people are consuming these foods. Until these issues are more adequately evaluated, street food vending in America might best be described as a melting pot; those who buy and sell food on the street are as diverse as the street foods themselves.

Conclusion

There has been a dynamic change in the street food vending industry in the United States. Whereas the industry started with single carts offering predominantly one food (i.e. ice cream or hot dogs), it is now characterized by carts that offer a variety of foods including many different ethnic foods that are popular in specific locales. Consequently, the consumer is confronted with many food choices ranging from snack foods to sandwiches and other meal items that can be eaten simply as a snack or comprise an entire meal. As the street food vending industry has grown in certain cities and clearly has impacted the diets of many consumers, there is the realization that we have little information about the contribution of these foods to the American diet. Specifically, we know little about the contribution of street foods to the energy and nutrient intake of US consumers. Furthermore, little is known about the food behavior practices of people who patronize street food vendors. Thus, we need to understand the patterns of street food consumption (i.e. frequency, type and amount) and how they affect other food choice behaviors. This information will be invaluable in identifying nutrition education needs of consumers who purchase street foods. This will facilitate the development of nutrition education programs for the street food industry. The goal should be to have this information available at the point-of-purchase of street foods so that consumers can make informed food choices and, thereby, plan healthy diets.

References

1   New York Times, March 30, 1930, as noted in reference 2.
2   Bluestone D: The pushcart evil; in Ward D, Zunz O (ed): Landscape of Modernity. New York, Russell Sage Foundation, 1992, pp 287–312.
3   Wright R: Hawkers and Walkers in Early America. Philadelphia, Lippincott, 1927, pp 233–234, as noted in reference 2.
4   Manhattan Borough President of John Purroy Mitchel, ca Sept 1914, Mayor John P Mitchel Papers, Box 215, New York City Municipal Archives, as noted in reference 2.
5   The Picture of New York and Stranger's Guide to the Commercial Metropolis of the United States. New York, AT Goodrich, 1828, pp 425–426, as noted in reference 2.
6   Gartner LP: The Jews of New York's east side, 1890–1893: Two surveys by the Baron de Hirsch Fund. Am Jewish Q 1964;53:265–285.
7   French ER: Push Cart Markets in New York City (US Department of Agriculture, Agricultural Economics Bureau and the Port of New York Authority, March, 1925), pp 34–35, as noted in reference 2.
8   French ER: Push Cart Markets in New York City (US Department of Agriculture, Agricultural Economics Bureau and the Port of New York Authority, March, 1925), p 7, as noted in reference 2.
9   Hamilton LJ to Morgan WF Jr, June 30, 1938: LaGuardia Papers, New York City Municipal Archives, as noted in reference 2.
10 Commissioner Albert S. Pacetta: New York City Department of Markets, Annual Report for the Year Ending 30 June 1964, pp 43–44, as noted in reference 2.

11 Trager J: The Food Chronology: A Food Lover's Compendium of Events, Anecdotes, from Prehistory to the Present. New York, Henry Holt, 1995.

12 Louie E: A savory guide to the exotica of Chinatown's food vendors. New York Times, June 16, 1993, p Cl.

13 Dubner S: Street Treats. New York, December 23, 1991, pp 96–97.

14 Lin B-H, Frazazo E: Nutritional quality of foods at and away from home. Food Review, May-August 1997, pp 33–40.

15 WHO: Essential Safety Requirements for Street-Vended Foods. Geneva, WHO, 1996.

16 Drummond KE: Nutrition for the Food Service Professional. New York, Van Nostrand Reinhold, 1997, p 136.

17 Abdussalam M, Kaferstein FK: Safety of street foods. Wld Hlth Forum 1993;14:191–194.

18 New York State Department of Health: A review of foodborne disease outbreaks in New York State: 1992 and 1993. New York State Department of Health, 1996.

19 Bryan FL: Risks associated with vehicles of foodborne pathogens and toxins. J Food Prot 1988; 51:498–508.

20 Bean NH, Griffin PM: Foodborne disease outbreaks in the United States, 1973–1987: Pathogens, vehicles, and trends. J Food Prot 1990;53:804–817.

21 Bean NH, Goulding JS, Daniels MT, Angulo FJ: Surveillance for foodborne disease outbreaks – United States, 1988–1992. J Food Prot 1997;60:1265–1286.

22 Todd ECD: Foodborne and Waterborne Disease in Canada, Annual Summaries, 1985 and 1986. Ottawa, Health Protection Branch, Health & Welfare Canada, 1991.

23 Todd ECD: Foodborne disease in Canada: A 10-year summary from 1975–1984. J Food Prot 1992; 55:123–132.

24 WHO Technical Report Series, No 705: The role of food safety in health and development: Report of the joint FAO/WHO Expert Committee on Food Safety. Geneva, WHO, 1984.

25 Bryan FL, Standley SR, Henderson WC: Time-temperature conditions of gyros. J Food Prot 1980; 43:346–353.

26 Bryan FL, Bartleson CA, Christopherson N: Hazard analyses, in reference to *Bacilllus cereus*, of boiled and fried rice in Cantonese-style restaurants. J Food Prot 1981;44:500–512.

27 Bryan FL, Bartleson CA, Sugi M, Sakai B, Miyashiro L, Tsutsumi S, Chun C: Hazard analysis of *char siu* and roast pork in Chinese restaurants and markets. J Food Prot 1982;45:422–429.

28 Bryan FL, Sugi M, Miyashiro L, Tsutsumi S, Bartleson CA Hazard analysis of duck in Chinese restaurants. J Food Prot 1982;45:445–449.

29 Bryan FL, Michanie S, Alvarez P, Paniagua A: Critical control points of street-vended foods in the Dominican Republic. J Food Prot 1988;51:373–384.

30 Bryan FL, Fukunaga I, Tsutsumi S, Miyashiro L, Kagawa D, Sakai B, Matsuura, H, Oramura M: Hazard analysis of Japanese boxed lunches (bento). J Environ Health 1991;54:29–32.

31 Bryan FL, Teufel P, Riaz S, Roohi S, Qadar F, Malik Z: Hazards and critical control points of vending operations at a railway station and a bus station in Pakistan. J Food Prot 1992;55:534–541.

32 Bryan FL, Teufel P, Riaz S, Roohi S, Qadar F, Malik Z: Hazards and critical control points of street-vending operations in a mountain resort town in Pakistan. J Food Prot 1992;55:701–707.

33 Bryan FL, Teufel P, Roohi S, Qadar F, Riaz S, Malik Z: Hazards and critical control points of street-vended *chat*, a regionally-popular food in Pakistan. J Food Prot 1992;55:708–713.

34 El-Sherbeeny MR, Saddik MF, Aly HE-S, Bryan FL: Microbiological profile and storage temperatures of Egyptian rice dishes. J Food Prot 1985;48:39–43.

35 El-Sherbeeny MR, Saddik MF, Bryan FL: Microbiological profiles of foods sold by street vendors in Egypt. Int J Food Microbiol 1985;2:355–364.

36 New York State Department of Health, Bureau of Community Sanitation and Food Protection: Chapter 1, State Sanitary Code. Subpart 14-4, Mobile Food Service Establishments/Foodcarts (Statutory Authority: Public Health Law §224). January 8, 1997.

37 Gaber J: Manhattan's 14th street vendors' market: Informal street peddlers' complementary relationship with New York City's economy. Urban Anthropol 1994;23:373–408.

38 Pan PP: Honorable work or illegal activity? In Langley Park, its 'Pupusa ladies' vs county agencies, with Latino officers caught in middle. Washington Post, August 24, 1997, p B3.

39   Ginsburg J: City cracks down on mobile food vendors. Chicago Tribune, July 27, 1991, p 5.
40   Editorial: A muddled policy on food vendors. New York Times, June 13, 1994, p A14.
41   Editorial: Still fighting over food vendors. New York Times, September 30, 1995, p A18.
42   Tinker I: Street Foods. Urban Food and Employment in Developing Countries. New York, Oxford University Press, 1997.
43   Moy G, Hazzard A, Kaferstein F: Improving the safety of street-vended food. World Health Stat Q 1997;50:124–131.
44   Spalter-Roth RM: The sexual, political economy of street vending in Washington, DC; in Spalter-Roth RM, Zeitz B (eds): Street Vending in Washington, DC: Reassessing the Regulation of a 'Public Nuisance'. Washington, George Washington University, 1985, pp 165–187.
45   National Restaurant Association: Off-Premises Market. Washington, NRA, 1993.

P.M. Kris-Etherton, Nutrition Department, The Pennsylvania State University,
S-126 Henderson Building, University Park, PA 16802 (USA)
Tel. +1 (814) 863 2923, Fax +1 (814) 863 6103

Simopoulos AP, Bhat RV (eds): Street Foods.
World Rev Nutr Diet. Basel, Karger, 2000, vol 86, pp 45–52

....

Public (Street) Foods in Australia

Mark Wahlqvist [a], *Anthony Worsley* [b], *Ingrid Flight* [a]

[a] International Health and Development Unit, Faculty of Medicine,
Monash University, Melbourne, Victoria, and
[b] Department of Public Health, University of Adelaide, Australia

The concept of street or public foods is rarely seen as being a part of developed countries such as Australia with its 5,400 supermarkets and 130,000 other retail food establishments [1] serving a population of approximately 18 million people. Street foods tend to be viewed by the casual observer as having more to do with the bazaars and markets of developing countries in Asia, Africa and Latin America. However, we would argue that many foods are available and consumed in public places in Australia and other western countries. The variety and consumption of such 'public foods' remain relatively unexplored perhaps because of the assumption that most foods consumed in industrialised countries must be solely delivered by industrial production and distribution systems. In this brief overview we wish to draw attention to the existence of this broad category of food consumption which is entrenched within Australian cultural contexts.

The review is indicative rather than exhaustive because little information has been reported in either the scholarly or business literatures. Most information, particularly about sales figures, has been collected by commercial sources who regard it as 'commercial in confidence' and so are loath to put it into the public domain.

What Are Public Foods?

We prefer the term 'public foods' to 'street foods' since the locations of supply and consumption are more varied than the street, e.g. sports grounds, church fetes, shopping malls, cinemas. By 'public foods' we refer to the immediate purchase and consumption of ready-to-eat foods in public places. Public foods have an element of environmental proximity about them which require little anticipation, planning or preparation on the part of the consumer. They form part of the class of convenience foods but are purchased and usually consumed in a public location – though some foods are undoubtedly purchased for later consumption in the home, e.g. jams, preserved fruit and cakes from church and other fetes. They are part of a rising trend in Australian and other western societies, the fast food or convenience food trend [2].

Various estimates have been made of the proportions of meals which are prepared outside the home; between a quarter and one third of meals appear to fall into this category. BIS Shrapnel in their report *The Australian Food Service Market* (1997) claim that within 20 years half of all food expenditure will be for meals prepared outside the home. Sandwiches, hot chips (french fries) and hamburgers were rated as the three most popular takeaway products in 1995, followed by cakes, filled rolls, pizzas and doughnuts. In a later report, *Fast Food in Australia 1995–1997*, the same market research company estimated that there are now over 16,000 fast food and takeaway outlets in Australia. Supermarkets, greengrocers and butchers' shops are responding to this trend through the provision of 'ready to eat', 'ready to heat' and 'oven ready' meat kiosks, and fresh convenience foods. Around 39% of the retail and commercial food service market in 1996 comprised takeaway and fast food products.

Public foods appear to have emerged or re-emerged along with convenience foods, ready to eat, pre-prepared, foods, take away foods, oven ready foods, dash board foods, as-you-go foods, and similar categories coined by marketers.

The social economic constraints which have influenced this extra-domestic source of foods have not been examined in much detail. Food industry observers generally associate the rise of convenience foods to the growth in the married female permanent work force during the past 40 years [2]. In turn, changes in social and economic policy such as the abolition of tax benefits for families with children may also have partly influenced this trend [3]. However, the purchase and consumption of public foods has a much longer history reaching back into Australia's urban and rural roots in Europe, Asia and elsewhere.

Types of Public Foods

The types of public foods available in Australia can be thought of in terms of their geographic and cultural contexts mainly within urban areas (since Australia, despite its huge land area, is a highly urbanised country).

Foods Sold at Agricultural and Horticultural Shows and Fair Grounds
Most Australian States and territories have annual agricultural shows (Royal Shows) which are mirrored in country towns. These shows may last for

up to a week and include displays of domestic and farm animals, agricultural machinery and skills (e.g. wood chopping exhibitions, floral arrangement competitions), side show alleys (fun fares). The sale of 'show bags', filled mainly with confectionery products is a traditional feature. Many people visit these events, for example, the Royal Adelaide Show attracts around 600,000 people out of a total State population of 1.4 million of these shows.

The foods available include fish and chips (french fries), hot chips in a cardboard bucket (french fries), hamburgers, meat pies, cornish pasties, hot dogs, candy floss, super dogs (sausage on a stick), chiko rolls (large fried spring rolls, derivative of Chinese cuisine), sausage and onion rolls, steak sandwiches, dim sims (a Chinese mixed pork and flour encased snack which may be steamed or fried), ice cream, iced confectionery, waffles, doughnuts, confectionery products, flavoured milks, tea, coffee, spring and mineral water, cola, carbonated and alcoholic beverages, among others. Nutrition consciousness is not apparent among Show patrons.

Foods Sold at Sporting Events

These include cricket, netball, football and many other sporting fixtures such as horse trials, rodeos, and motor car racing. The range of foods sold by small traders, who are usually licensed by local authorities, is similar to that described above. Again large numbers of people and large amounts of food may be involved. For example, at the Adelaide Grand Prix (motor racing) in 1991 175,000 litres of soft drink, 150,000 hot dogs, 250,000 ice creams, 3,000 kg of seafood, 16,000 kg of cold meats, and 2,500 kg of fresh fruit were sold to total patronage approximately 100,000 people [Chong, Adelaide City Council, pers. commun.]. At Australian Rules football matches, it is a custom to eat meat pies (filled with minced beef and gravy) with plentiful amounts of tomato sauce.

Foods Sold at Places of Entertainment

Cinemas and theatres are traditional locations for the sale and consumption of a limited range of foods, mainly consisting of pop corn, ice cream products, and carbonated drinks. In some cities, sporting clubs and gambling establishments are also associated with a variety of foods. In New South Wales, 'leagues clubs' associated with Rugby league clubs have large memberships accounting for much of the adult population. They are renowned for the provision of inexpensive meals (supplemented through gambling revenues from poker machines 'one armed bandits'). They generally serve simple cooked meals consisting of meat (e.g. 'schnitzel'), vegetables such as carrots, pumpkin, salads and hot chips. However, extensive ranges of meals are served in some establishments. Strictly these are not public foods since they are served and consumed on private premises but they do form part of the common lifestyle of many Australians. In the past decade the spread of legalised gambling has seen a proliferation of 'pub foods' in Victoria, South Australia and elsewhere.

A notable feature in certain entertainment districts of Australian cities is the mobile 'pie cart' (mobile food vendors) which typically operate late at night, serving meat pies, pasties, hamburgers, and non-alcoholic beverages. Close to the Adelaide casino, an updated version of a traditional pie cart serves what most South Australians recognise as authentic local cuisine – the 'pie floater' a meat pie floating face down in a bowl of pea soup, topped with tomato sauce! For many this dish symbolises their State identity.

Formal Food Fairs

One in four adult Australians were born abroad, many of them in Mediterranean and Asian countries. The result has been an explosion in the diversity of foods available in the country since World War Two. From time to time during the year street celebrations of ethnic identity are held throughout the country, for example in South Australia Cornish Festivals are held in the old mining towns of the northern Yorke Peninsula; German Festivals are held in the wine growing Barossa Valley; and the annual Glendi (Greek) Festival is held in Adelaide, and Chinese New Year celebrations are to be found in Melbourne and other towns and cities. Foods associated with one or more ethnicities are sold and consumed during these festivities.

Similarly, local city councils may regularly organise local food fairs where a range of meals from diverse cuisines are available for sale and consumption. There are opportunities for researchers to document the ways in which public foods reflect the ethnic and cultural traditions of Australia's population. Subtle differences in the food consumption of the population of various cities has been reported [National Nutrition Survey, 1997]. These may well reflect the historical traditions of both indigenous and immigrants to the various States and they may be exhibited in the types of publicly available foods.

A good example is the Unley City Council in South Australia which runs the Unley Dine and Wine event. The aim of organisers is to attract customers to local food service businesses. Local restaurants combine to offer a number of meals and wines in the centre of the local sporting oval for a set fee. They rent the places for a fee from the council. Typical meals include teppanyaki, teriyaki, chicken breast with pearl barley and wild rice, asparagus in pastry, tandoori, Malay dishes, Chinese dishes and more. These are gourmet foods rather than 'fast foods' but nevertheless they are a fairly typical though small part of the Australian public food scene. At the perimeter of the Unley Oval there are around 100 booths (also rented from the council) which are run by community groups, about half of them offer food such as chops and sausages.

The most popular food is sausage in bread with sauce. The remaining food stalls sell home-made cakes, jams, biscuits, ice cream, and occasionally, pancakes. About 10,000 people attend the Festival over the course of the day.

Whilst most the food vendors at these events are locals licensed by the local council two other kinds of sellers often appear. One group is the 'sideshow professionals' who sells foods such as hot potatoes and Copenhagen ice cream – they have to pay a higher price for their booths as they are not locals. The other type of vendor is the 'fast food hijacker' who sneaks in unannounced, parks his/her mobile food vehicle by the children's area and sells foods such as ice creams and waffles. By the time a council official notices them occupying a place which has not been paid for, there is usually a long queue of children who would be most upset if the vendor was asked to move away!

Mobile ice cream vendors (e.g. Mr. Whippy) represent the remainder of a class of food vending which was popular in the mid century. This was the provision of groceries and greengroceries via mobile vans in large housing estates which had few shops.

'Informal' Food Fairs

A typical weekend event is a visit to a church or school or community 'fete'. Members of these community groups may combine on one or more occasions each year to prepare food and other products for sale to the local community. For example, members of a church congregation may set up a 'trading table' each month and sell foods such as jams, chutneys (pickled vegetables), cakes, and confectionery prepared by their members, usually by their older members (aged 60 years or older). Typically, they raise about $A 250 for church projects. The same congregation conducts an annual fete and a Christmas Festival. On these occasions, a BBQ is provided (serving sausages in bread and tomato sauce) [Rev. M. Bowers, St Augustine's Church, pers. commun.]. According to custom, Australian BBQs are cooked by men. They usually include the grilling of steaks and onions as well as sausages.

Less formal provision of foods may been seen at flea markets, trash and treasure and car boots sales usually held at weekends. Again, fast foods such as hot chips, pies, pasties, ice cream, tea and coffee are popular.

Food Markets and Fruit and Vegetable Stalls

Most Australian cities have large food markets where wholesalers, stall holders and the general public interact. A good example is the Victoria market in Melbourne. This opens to the public on several days each week. It supplies a wide variety of seafood, dairy products, fresh fruit and vegetables, and delicatessen products to the public, many of whom eat whilst they shop for clothing, toys and other manufactured goods.

Extension of this market culture can be observed in the mainstreet of many towns and cities in the form of mobile fruit and vegetable (and floral) vendors. Customers can buy one or two pieces of fruit for immediate consumption, or more for household meals.

Vending Machines

Vending machines provide a limited variety of foods and beverages at a number of public sites in Australia. For example, Smith Snack Vending has about 1,000 machines in the country in a number of locations including railway stations, bus stops, hotels, hospitals, recreational premises, as well as industrial, commercial and educational premises. The main customers are aged between 14 and 35 years. About 60% of the contents of the machines are snack foods such as crisps, the remainder are confectionery products [Luders, Smith Snack Vending, pers. commun.].

Vending machines can provide foods and drinks 'within an arms length of desire'. They are powerful ways to distribute certain classes of products. They can provide products 24 h a day in areas that are not serviced by shops, though often they are installed at the exits to shopping malls. For example, in Adelaide alone, Coca Cola Amatil has about 4,500 beverage vending machines, 850 of them in public thoroughfares – all of the latter have been installed within the past 2 years. Further expansion of machines in public places is proposed. Australians are the third highest consumers of carbonated beverages after Americans and Mexicans. However, vendor penetration is only one third that of the USA because of a less-well-developed vending network. [Fitzgerald Coca Cola Amatil, pers. commun.]. Beverages provided by the vending machines include Coca Cola, Fanta, Sprite, Diet Coke, carbonated fruit drinks and mineral waters. Women tend to prefer carbonated fruit drinks and diet Coke, men prefer Coca Cola, Fanta and Sprite.

A recent development which blurs the distinction between public foods and shop food is the sale of fast food products from petrol service stations. BP Australia developed a network of 'BP Express' convenience stores which emphasise bakery and pizza products. The food section consists of a central island with refrigeration and heating facilities. The bakery sells such items as: Danish pastries, croissants, muffins, and breads. The facilities also sell chicken rolls, sandwiches, pizzas, hamburgers, 'hound dogs' (hot dogs), pies and pasties and well as soft drinks, and fruit juices. The main market in the morning up to 2 p.m. is for sandwiches, which are mostly sold to blue collar workers. More pizzas, burgers, hound dogs, pies and pasties are sold in the afternoon, mostly to young people around 14–25 years of age [Senior, BP Australia, pers. commun.].

Who Uses Public Foods?

Little is known about the consumers of public foods. It is known that teenagers and young people tend to make greater use of vending machine foods and snack foods provided through petrol stations (as described above). Although some industry data (from BP Australia) suggests that blue collar workers purchase more snack foods this cannot be regarded as typical of the general community. Indeed, Santich's [4] analysis of the Australian Household expenditure survey suggest that affluent families are greater consumers of fast foods than poorer families. Similar, gender and age group preferences remain unknown at present. There is a need for more research in this area.

Nutritional and Food Safety Aspects of Public Foods

Brief consideration of the most popular public foods (e.g. hot chips, hamburgers, pies, ice cream, carbonated beverages) might suggest that they are not of the greatest nutritional quality being in the main high-fat, high-sugar, low dietary fibre foods. However, before any judgement of nutritional appropriateness can be made, the place of these foods in the consumers' diets needs to be assessed. Unfortunately, at present little information is available about the population's consumption of these foods and those from other sources. The recent National Nutrition Survey, for example, does not provide information about the source of foods.

Anecdotally, however, in clinical practice one of us (M.W.) has confirmed industry observations that some adolescents and young single people appear to consume large amounts of public foods. Some individuals may consume little else. It may well be that for some individuals these foods may be important sources of a variety of nutrients (e.g. vitamins, minerals) which they would not otherwise consume. Research is required to decide whether these foods pose any serious threat to the health of the population, or indeed whether they are a source of valuable nutrients. However, in the absence of any estimates of the amounts of these foods that are consumed by the public further speculation is unwarranted.

A number of food safety issues are involved in public foods. These relate to unsupervised production and storage of foods, particularly dairy and meat products which are excellent media for a variety of organisms which can be responsible for foodborne illnesses. Outbreaks of foodborne illness are reported to environmental health authorities from time to time. Small manufacturers and suppliers of foods are believed to account for most of the burden of foodborne illness in Australia. Local councils attempt to prevent potential epidemics of foodborne illness through licensing of stall holders and vendors. However, resource limitations prevent inspections of the vast majority of vendors. Instead, vendors are issued with food safety guidelines, and refuse bins are usually provided by the local councils. The situation is likely to change in the near future with recommendations for compulsory food safety training for all food vendors in Australia (including Hazard Analysis Critical Control Points training promoted by the Australia and New Zealand Food Authority and the Food Safety Code in Victoria; for further details see http://hna.tth.vic.gov.au/phb/).

Conclusions

This brief overview has shown that public foods are an important but unexplored facet of Australians' food and nutrition. A major research effort is required to describe and quantify Australians' consumption of public foods and to examine some of the cultural, social and economic influences on their use of this class of foods.

References

1   Bevan B: How to beat McDonald's, KFC and the Pizza huts. Retail World 1995;48:8.
2   McKay H: Reinventing Australia. Sydney: Angus and Robertson of the food scene. Choice, December, 1994, pp 12–17.
3   Edgar DE: Conceptualising family life and family policies. Family Matters 1992;32:28–37.
4   Santich BJ: Socioeconomic status and consumption of snack and take-away foods. Food Aust 1995; 47:121–126.

Prof. Mark Wahlqvist, Asia Pacific Health and Nutrition Center, Monash Asia Institute,
8th Floor Manzies Building, Monash University, Wellington Road,
Clayton, Victoria 3168 (Australia)
Tel. +61 3 9905 8145, Fax +61 3 9905 8146, E-Mail mark.wahlqvist@med.monash.edu.au

Simopoulos AP, Bhat RV (eds): Street Foods.
World Rev Nutr Diet. Basel, Karger, 2000, vol 86, pp 53–99

....

Profile of Street Foods Sold in Asian Countries

Ramesh V. Bhat, Kavita Waghray

National Institute of Nutrition, Indian Council of Medical Research,
Hyderabad, India

History

The proliferation of street foods in Asian countries is a recent phenomenon and has a history of only about 5–6 decades. In India, during olden days because of the strong caste system, eating foods prepared by persons of another caste were forbidden. Despite this, on some occasions like local festivals, and shandies, street food vending was in vogue. The concept of street foods in a modern sense started way back in the 1940s. Near the schools, vendors used to sell ice creams, ice balls and foods like 'churan' and 'bajji' (onion green chilli). In the summer months, mobile vendors used to sell 'kulfi' traditional sweet in the late evenings. Analysis of the quality parameters of ice creams started from early forties and standards fixed for ice creams [1].

Street foods were observed in Khatmandu, Nepal over the past 50 years. During those days the street foods were Chatamari (prepared from rice flour), Phulaura (prepared from wheat and broad bean flour), gulfuki (salted puffed rice) and roasted corn, beaten rice, etc. Seasonal fruits and root vegetables (boiled potatoes, sweet potatoes, raddish) were also available in the market as ready to eat foods [2]. During the period between 1970 and 1980 items like cakes, pastries, different types of breads (loafs and doughnuts), Tibetan foods as Mamacha (prepared from wheat dough stuffed with minced meat) noodles and also Indian foods like samosa, chhole, bahture, etc., along with varieties of meat cooked, boiled, fried, roasted, minced and spicy raw meat were popular. The Tibetan foods were generally taken along with alcoholic drinks rather than tea and coffee. Tea was available only the last 30 years. Even until 20 years back, there were a few items sold on the streets patronized mostly by the poor people [2].

The inexpensive medley of culinary delights provided by the ubiquitous street food hawkers in Malaysia goes back to the time when the early Chinese traders came to Penang to trade with the Malays. Then came the Indians who brought in not only their trade but also their culture and tradition including their food and methods of preparation. This multiracial factor served as the main contribution to the availability of an endless selection of food in Malaysia [3].

In the 1950s and 1960s street hawkers were a common sight in Singapore. Many people took up hawking as means of making a living. It was a way out for the unemployed. By late 1960s however, the unemployment situation improved with rapid industrial and economic developments. The hawker population had grown in great proportion by 1968 and measures were taken to prevent further proliferation of street hawkers. The government conducted island-wide census of street hawkers in 1968–1969 which indicated the existence of 18,000 street hawkers. Those registered in the census were issued temporary street hawking licenses. Hawking activities in the streets, however, were unhygienic and led to pollution. There was no direct water supply and food wastes were indiscriminately discharged into open drains. They also caused obstruction to pedestrian and vehicular traffic. Hence, in 1971 the government decided to build markets and food centers to relocate street hawkers. These markets and food centers were provided with amenities and infrastructures to enable hawkers to conduct their business under clean and hygienic conditions, direct water and electricity supplies and disposal and pollution control facilities were provided [4]. Street food vendors in Taiwan have probably existed for hundreds of years [5].

Socioeconomic Aspects

Employment
In the Asian continent street food industry is a vast business involving huge amounts of monies and millions of people [6]. It is an activity that provides employment to large sectors of population (both skilled or unskilled) which might otherwise be unemployed [7]. It employs 6–25% of the work force sometimes involving entire families. It also provides outlets for utilization of agricultural and other produce [8]. Battcock [9] and Wedgewood et al. [10] reported that in urban areas of Bangladesh street food business employs over 6% of the work force while in Bogor (Indonesia) roughly 26% of workers active in the informal sector were directly or indirectly involved in the street food industry [11, 12]. Studies conducted in Penang (Malaysia) revealed that the street food sector has generated as much as 20,000 jobs or 12% of the

Table 1. Total sales of street food in selected Asian countries

Country	Annual turnover	Year	Ref. No.
Bangladesh	USD 2 million	1992, 1994	9, 10
China	20 billion Chinese yuan	1992	7
India	USD 60 million	1996	18
Malaysia	USD 2.2 billion	1988	19
Philippines (Iloilo)	USD 28 million	1986	15

total employment on the island [3]. Another study conducted by Aziz [13] revealed that street food vendors generated about 40,000 jobs. Two studies conducted in Iloilo city (Philippines) revealed that 18–26% of the urban labor force derived their income from street food sales [14, 15].

Economics

The contribution of street food vendors to the economics of Asian countries has been vastly underestimated and neglected and the available information is summarized in table 1 [16, 17].

Food Budget Spent

In Asia urban households 15–50% of their food budgets were spent on street foods [15]. Studies carried out in Indonesia and Malaysia indicated that the food budget spent on street food was a quarter of the total budget while in Philippines and Singapore it was almost 1/3 of the total budget [12, 20]. Customer surveys in the Asian countries indicate that street foods are consumed by the people in all income groups [21]. Many people in Asia prefer to make frequent small purchases at convenient locations. Those with little or no income depend almost exclusively on food supplied by street food vendors. Street foods are a bargain for customers when the demands of time and costs of food, fuel, cooking equipment, and transportation are taken into account [19, 22].

Amongst the lower income groups, in several developing countries 50–70% of their earnings go on food. However, it would be wrong to assume that only poor or low income people eat street foods. On the contrary, because of the variety of foods offered, almost all segments of society visit street food vendors [23]. Income spent on street food by different categories of people varied from place to place (table 2).

In Thailand where multiple dishes are the traditional diet, 70% of the households in Chonburi do not cook food for every meal and thus depend

Table 2. Percentage of income spent on street foods in Asian countries

Country	City	Income spent on street foods %	Year	Ref. No.
Bangladesh	Manikgunj	16	1986	15
India	Anantapur	50	1993	24
India	Secunderabad	10–15	1990	25
India	Pune	6.6–14	1986	26
Indonesia	Bogor	63	1991	16
Philippines	Iloilo	28	1986	15
Thailand	Bangkok	50	1994	27
Thailand	Chonburi	47	1987	28

on the street foods eaten on site or brought home. Around 13% of those surveyed never cook at home, many are government employees who were transferred to town and have left their wives and families elsewhere. Households where wives work away from home spend somewhat more for street foods than those households where the wife stays home. One of the busiest times of day is late afternoon as working wives pick up their families' evening meals, the vendors call them 'plastic bag housewives' [28].

Recent trends in countries like Malaysia and India have indicated that the percentage of income devoted to the purchase of street food declines as income rises and the strength of the eating out tradition is also a key variable affecting the level of street foods demand and amount spent which is low in Bangladesh and high in other Southeast Asian countries [15].

Franchise

In Asian countries, a large number of street food businesses were set up by various groups of people after receiving money from different sources like loans from banks, own savings, friends and relatives, advance from multinational companies, moneylenders, voluntary associations such as NAESEY (National Association of Educated Self-Employed Youth), and cooperatives. The majority of the enterprises in India (88–97%) are started with own savings, while the rest have help from banks (3.8%), relatives (4.4%), or cooperatives (3.6%). In contrast, the source of money was mostly from relatives in Bangladesh (80%), the Philippines (65%) and Thailand (36%) [25–29].

The number of persons involved in street food businesses varies from country to country in Asia and ranges from 1 to 6. The average number of persons per establishment was between 1.5 and 2 in Bangladesh and Indonesia

[15], between 2 and 3 in Hyderabad (India) [30], Pakistan [31], and Iloilo, Philippines [15, 28], and between 1 and 6 in Secunderabad, India [25] and Bangkok, Thailand [27].

Cost of Street Foods

The cost of street foods varied from vendor to vendor depending upon the nature of the customers and area in which he is catering to. Studies conducted in Calcutta revealed that the cost of street foods ranged from Rs. 0.50–8 per serving (1 USD = 39 Rs.) which was lower when compared to the cost of most modest restaurants [32]. Similar observations were also made in Hyderabad, Parbhani and Pune. The cost of different snack preparations sold by vendors in Hyderabad ranged from Rs. 0.75 to 3.50 [30]. While in Parbhani the cost per 100 g of snack preparation ranged from Rs. 1 to 4 [33] and in Pune the cost per 100 g snack ranged from Rs. 0.80 to 5. The meal side dishes cost Rs. 0.86 to 3.53, frozen foods Rs. 2 to 4.60, drinks Rs. 0.40 to 3; sweet meats Rs. 1 to 3 and popular miscellaneous items (local seasonal foods) Rs. 0.80 to 2.40 [26].

Role of Women

Women play a dominant role in the street food industry. They play a major role not only in the preparation and serving of the street foods but also in the marketing. Studies conducted in various Asian countries have shown a range in the employment of women in the street food preparations of 1–90% [6]. The percentage of women engaged in the street food trade was only 1% in Manikgunj (Bangladesh), 14% in Bogor, <30% in Nepal and some parts of Indonesia, 75% in Chonburi (Thailand), and 90% in Iloilo (Philippines) [15, 21, 23, 28]. In contrast, in countries like India and Bangladesh, it was male dominated and the percentage of male vendors ranged from 90 to 99% [9, 26, 30, 34].

According to Hutabarat [27] in Bangkok 69.3% of women were owners with 73.85% of their employees being females. Thus, the women outnumbered men 2 to 1. All the employees in the ambulatory street food business were females. Even in countries such as Bangladesh where the sellers of street food were men, a quarter of the street vendors were found to have had help with food preparation at home by their wives and 12% employed female helpers. In Bogor (Indonesia) women were often relieved of their home tasks by other family members [35]. Most of the foods women made were fairly traditional. There were also some indications that women had less access to new foodstuffs. For example, in Bogor (Indonesia) women made rice-based sweet dishes while men made wheat-based dishes, like breads and noodles [36, 37]. Most of the traditional rice-based sweets in Indonesia and many of the fried lentils and puffed rice snacks in Bangladesh were made by women working alone or in groups.

There is some sex specificity in the mode of selling of street foods. Women were selling out of baskets which could be carried on one's head while no woman was observed pushing a mobile cart. In some cases in Jakarta men pushed the cart into place each morning and removed it at night for their wives [38]. Women sold nearly all types of food though only a few women sold noodles exclusively and a few soup in Bogor (Indonesia) [39].

In Southeast Asia women vendors have been found to have flourishing businesses. Enterprises run by couples have the highest sales in countries like the Philippines and Indonesia. Couple enterprises are dominated by women in the Philippines. When successful women run enterprises which have grown enough to provide two incomes, the husband joins his wife in the business. The situation is reversed in Indonesia, women entrepreneurs have a slightly higher income than men. In both countries women vendors were found at all levels of the income scale [39].

In Chobnuri (Thailand) 20% of the women provided the main source of income for their families. While another 21% of the women vendors who were unmarried contributed to their families' income. In Bangladesh, all the women vendors (n = 5) were the sole income earners in their families [39]. In most of the Asian countries (e.g. Thailand, Philippines, Indonesia, Bangladesh), the woman's income was used for household expenditure and for school fees [28].

Profile of Street Vendors

The number of street food vendors varied from country to country on the Asian continent (table 3). This observation in the population of street food vendors was related to the total population, urbanization, and cultural habits. The ratio of vendors to the total population varied from 1:14 to 1:901 (table 3). In most of the countries the ratio was less than 1:500 except in Bangkok and Hyderabad where the ratios were very high, i.e. 1:901 and 1:800.

Age
Tinker [28] reported that in Manikgunj (Bangladesh), Chonburi (Thailand), Iloilo (Philippines) and Bogor (Indonesia), the average age of the vendors is 20–45 years. This shows consistency across the cultures. Another major observation in most Asian countries is that less than 5% of the vendors were children [18, 23, 26, 28, 30] aged less than 20 years. Waghray and Bhat [48] reported that during special exhibitions in Hyderabad, children (40 of 168 vendors) were involved with vending of street foods. In Bangkok city (Thai-

Table 3. Population/census of street food vendors and ratio of street food vendors to total population

Country	City/town	Total population	Total number of street vendors	Ratio	Ref. No.
Bangladesh	Manikgunj	38,000	550	1:69	21
China	Beijing	–	72,176	–	6
	8 districts	–	24,341		
	Liaoning Province (12 cities and 41 provinces)	–	32,692	–	40
	Shaanxi Province Yin Chaun city	–	>10,000	–	41
	Year 1988	–	489	–	42
	Year 1992	–	2,185	–	
	total	–	>1 million	–	6
India	Bombay	12,571,720	25,000	1:503	43
	Greater Calcutta	9,000,000	150,000	1:60	32
	Hyderabad	4,000,000	5,000	1:800	44
	Pune	–	1,382	–	45
Indonesia	Bogor	248,000	17,760	1:14	21, 17
Malaysia	Kuala Lumpur	11,690,591	28,478	1:41	46
	Penang	521,181	5,040	1:103	3
	total	–	40,434	–	7
Philippines	Iloilo city	244,827	5,100	1:48	28
Singapore	Singapore	26,000,000	23,331	1:111	4
Thailand	Bangkok metropolis	–	120,000	–	47
	135 municipalities of 72 provinces	–	20,000	–	47
	Bangkok	5,620,591	6,237	1:901	27
	Chonburi	46,000	950	1:48	21, 17
Vietnam	–	–	55,152	–	7

land), the average age of owners of street food business was 36 years while that of employees was 27 years. Owners, whether male or female, were considerably older than their employees [27].

Educational Level

Education also varies across the sample. Illiteracy is presumed to characterize vendors. It is also true among the women vendors in the more traditional

Islamic countries (e.g. Bangladesh). In Manikgunj (Bangladesh) all women vendors were illiterate. However, the male vendors had considerable schooling with only 32% illiterate, 26% with between 6 and 10 years of school and another 6% with vocational school training [28]. Chen et al. [5] reported that in Henan Province (China) only 22% of the food vendors had primary school education while 13.2% were illiterate.

A pilot study on improving the safety of urban street foods in some areas of five cities revealed that most of the street food vendors in Shaanxi Zhejiang and Lianing Provinces in China had a relatively low level of education on the whole. More than 85% of 2,009 vendors had less than junior middle school education, 22.2% had less than primary school. Around 14.8% were senior middle school graduates while 7.8% were illiterate [49].

Educational level of vendors varied from place to place in India. The majority were illiterate and few were university graduates. For example, in Calcutta (India), most of the vendors had primary level education and 21% were illiterate [18, 32]. In Chandigarh (India), most of the street food vendors were fairly well educated, i.e. up to junior secondary standard [50]. Bharathi [30] reported that in Hyderabad 46% were illiterate, 36% had secondary school education, while 18% had primary school education. In Pune almost 75.4% of the street food vendors did not complete primary school. Only 22.2% had completed secondary school education, while 2.2% were university graduates [26].

In Indonesia, the average schooling for street food vendors was elementary school or less. Almost 90% of the vendors had completed or at least attended elementary school, while the remaining 10% had undergone secondary level education [23]. Aziz [13] reported that in Malaysia the overall level of education was low with more than 50% of the food handlers having received only primary education till the age of 11 years and 23% of the managers having never been to school but the majority of this group had more than 5 years' experience in the food business. This possibly reflects the presence of traditional expertise, habits, beliefs and practices that are deep rooted and passed down from generation to generation, which may be contrary to modern practices of good food handling.

In Southeast Asia, both women and men had more education. For example, in Iloilo (Philippines), in contrast, the average education among the vendors was 8 years in school while 47% had 6 years or less, a third had completed high school, and 20% had some university education. Since Iloilo is a university town, some of the students who worked their way through college assisting street food vendors find that their income in this occupation is higher than most low-level governmental posts [28]. The educational background of street owners and employees in Bangkok (Thailand) ranged between no education at all to those who were university graduates. It was found that 49.8% of owners and 20% of employees had completed their education up to the elementary level. It was further found that 7–9% of owners and 6.8% of employees had never attended any formal education not even a short course [27]. Among the 247 street food handlers in Yin Chaun city (China), 19.44% had primary school education and 19.44% were illiterate [51].

Migration

Street food vendors were not recent migrants in any of the cities of Bangladesh, Indonesia, Philippines, or Thailand. Even among those who were not born in the town, most had lived there over 10 years. Many of those vendors born in rural areas near the city continue to live there and commute daily to work in the city. The pattern of migration into Bogor clearly reflects changes in the countryside and in this regard seems to fit the expected pattern of accelerating rural migration. The surge of migrants coincides with the introduction of a green revolution in rice cultivation, a system which requires fewer farm laborers. In Bogor, more women vendors (61%) than men (42%) were local in origin. This is the reverse of Chonburi (Thailand) where 80% of the men in contrast with only 33% of the women were native born [28].

Income

The street food vendors are attracted to the occupation because of the possibility of earning relatively high incomes [16]. In Southeast Asia, the average earnings of a vendor may be three to ten times more than the minimum wage and they are often comparable to the wages of skilled laborers employed in the formal sector. However, there is a wide variation between countries and within occupations. In many urban areas of Bangladesh, the street food business employs over 6% of the work force [9, 10]. The daily net income of a street vendor in Manikgunj (Bangladesh) (approximately 77 thaka) is three times more than that of the daily agricultural workers, more than twice the wage of an unskilled agricultural worker, more than that of a mason and about the equivalent of a carpenter [15, 28]. Similar observations were also made in India, for example, in Calcutta the income was between Rs. 1,500 and 4,000 [18]. In Pune (India), the average income for most street food vendors (62.7%) was between Rs. 1,000 and 3,000 per month; 11.4% earned Rs. 3,000–5,000 per month, while 15.6% earned above Rs. 5,000 per month which is above the average income of workers engaged in various factories. In Bogor (Indonesia) 50% of the street food vendors' daily net incomes were in the range of 1,700–3,100 rupiah, an income that is about twice the daily wage of construction workers [15]. In Malaysia also the net incomes of street food vendors varied from USD 4 to 36 (with an average of USD 16 per day) [52]. Another study conducted by Perdigon [3] revealed that the income of street food vendors in Penang (Malaysia) was M $65.50 per day for ambulant and stayput vendors. Average gross earnings of vendors in Iloilo (Philippines) were 54 pesos daily, which is again higher than that of a daily minimum formal sector unskilled wage earner – 33 pesos (a level of income only paid by registered, medium- and large-scale formal sector firms [15]. In Chonburi (Thailand), the daily income of the vendors ranged from 90 to 504 baht, with the lower end enough to support a family of 4–5 persons [15, 28]. The profits made by vendors near the government upper primary schools in the twin cities of Hyderabad and Secunderabad (India) varied from Rs. 5 to 35 per day [30, 53].

Number of Consumers Catered

Number of consumers catered by each vendor varied from place to place in the Asian countries. For example, Chakravarthy [32] reported that each vendor on average catered to approximately 65–70 customers per day in India. The number of customers varied at different times of the day, e.g. reaching a peak during the afternoon hours in office areas, and afternoons and evenings in shopping areas.

The proliferation of street foods is a fairly recent phenomenon in many Asian countries. In Chonburi (Thailand), the median length of street food enterprise was calculated as 7.2 years [28]. In Hyderabad (India), 84% of the vendors had been carrying out their operations for the last 5–10 years while in Calcutta the vendors had been operating for the last 1–10 years [18, 30]. In Manikgunj (Bangladesh) street food establishments have been in existence since the early 1960s.

Training

Several Asian countries do have an active training program administered by the government. In China, 68% of the street food vendors were qualified in food safety knowledge in urban areas and 46.9% in rural areas [49]. In contrast, in Calcutta (India) vendors had no basic training on safety of street foods. Health education in Singapore consists of periodic exhibitions, educational talks and slide shows, along with distribution of educational material such as posters and pamphlets. In the Philippines, Indonesia, training material has been designed and used for training food handlers in collaboration with local authorities. However, only a few countries have been involved in training programs and much remains to be done [6, 7, 54, 55]. Programs and strategies to improve all aspects of hawker food have been planned and implemented by various ministries and agencies such as the Ministry of Health, the Ministry of Local Government, and the Malaysian Agricultural Research Development Institute (MARDI) [7].

The Ministry of Health in Malaysia with the collaboration of other agencies has initiated programs such as the development of a curriculum for training of health inspectors on street food control, training of hawkers on sanitary and safe food preparation, preparing material and TV trailers. A massive relocation exercise as well as developing more practical facilities for street food preparation such as mobile kitchens has been undertaken by local authorities.

Personal Hygiene

Personal hygiene among the street vendors varied from place to place. Limited data have been collected by various researchers in this regard [12]. In Pune (India) the street vendor's knowledge and application of personal hygiene as well as food hygiene and sanitation was very much limited [26]. In Nepal, it was judged that 2% of the vendors 'looked' sick and 6.6% were dressed in dirty clothes [56].

Profile of Consumers

Limited data are available pertaining to the age group of consumers in the Asian countries though there is a wide variation in the age group ranging from preschool to 75 years. Out of 911 consumers interviewed in Calcutta 80% were males ranging in age from 17–48 years [18]. The majority of the consumers (n = 250) in Hyderabad (India) were aged less than 30 years (64.8%); 26% were between 30 and 40 years old and a few (4.4%) were between 40 and 60 years old. Almost 90% of them were aged below 40 years [30]. In Pune (India), similar observations were also made [26].

Unlike in other countries, in Indonesia and Thailand preschoolers were also regular consumers of street foods along with students (18–24 years) [15–16].

Educational Level

Very meager information is available regarding the educational level of the consumers. In Hyderabad (India) 56.4% of the consumers (n = 250) had higher education, 15.6% had secondary level; 13.6% had primary while 14.4% were illiterate [30].

Sex

In most of the Asian countries, the majority of the customers were males. For example, in Bangladesh 98% (n = 436) [28] and India, Hyderabad, 74.8% (n = 250) [30] were males and the rest were females. Unlike in Pune where both males and females were in equal proportions [26].

Table 4. Type of consumers patronizing street foods in Asian countries

Country	Type of consumer	Ref. No.
Bangladesh	rickshaw pullers, informal sector (43%), others (26%), white-collar workers (19%), children/students (12%), laborers	7, 21, 35 39
India		
Calcutta	low, middle high, high income group both sexes	18, 32
Coimbatore	elementary, high, higher secondary school and college students, adults	57
Hyderabad	students (32%), laborers (28.8%), businessmen (17.6%), housewives (20%)	30
Pune	businessmen, servicemen, workers, students (schools and college), housewives and others	26
Secunderabad	working class, businessmen (16.4%), servicemen (32.8%), workers (41.8%), students (4.3%), others (4.5%)	25
Indonesia		
Bogor	informal sector (37%), children/students (33%), others (16%), white-collar workers (14%)	18
Java and Sumatra	students of lower and middle socioeconomic class	12
Korea	urban workers	7
Nepal	poor people	7
Philippines		
Iloilo	informal sector (47%), white collar (21%), others (16%), children/students (16%)	18
Thailand		
Chonburi	informal sector (38%), white collar (20%), students/children (15%), housewives (10%), wage laborers (10%), others (7%)	18

Type of Consumer

The type of consumer of street foods varied from country to country on the Asian continent. They ranged from students to businessmen, to laborers, etc. Often they represent a broad spectrum of classes, viz. low, middle, high income groups (table 4).

Intake

Consumer intake of nutrients through street foods varied from place to place in Asia. In Indonesia, street foods like rice, fried fish and vegetables with egg supplemented for protein, and bread and tubers for calories are prevalent. All household members received an average of 14% of their calories,

Table 5. Frequency of consumption of street foods in Asian countries

Country/city	Frequency of consumption of street foods	Year	Ref. No.
India			
Calcutta	daily, 1–4 times/week (23%), occasionally	1996	18
Parbhani	4–5 times/day (70%), 2–3 times/day (30%)	1995	59
Pune	once to thrice a day	1986	26
Secunderabad	daily (37%), occasionally (4%), weekly (25%), monthly (4%), yearly (3%)	1990	25
Indonesia	3 meals/day (79%), 2 meals/day (18%)	1989	23

20% of their protein and 4% of their vitamin A from street foods [18]. In Bogor, more than half of the RDA of protein iron and vitamin A and vitamin C was acquired from a 30% street food meal [39]. In Hyderabad (India), males from a slum population consumed 600 kcal away from the home, a large part of which would have come from street foods [35], while in Bogor, among students 78% total energy intake, 82% total proteins and 79% iron intake were from street foods [58].

Hutabarat [27] reported that in Bangkok 44% of the energy intake for all sexes and age groups originated from street food. The greatest contribution by street food to daily energy intake was found in children aged 4–6 years (88%) followed by males aged 16–19 years (49%), females aged 20–29 years (48%) and females aged 30–39 years (42%). The same order of ranking was found with respect to protein, fat, carbohydrate and iron intakes.

The total daily energy intakes for the various occupational groups were 47% for farmers, 52% for skilled workers, 40% for students, 45% for housewives, 36% for teachers, 51% for government officials, and 42% for businessmen; higher compared to other sources. Similar observations were made with respect to protein, fat, carbohydrate and iron intakes.

Frequency

Frequency of consumption of street foods by the consumers varied from person to person (table 5). In Singapore, one million food meals are purchased every day and, on average, one street food meal is eaten daily by most adults [56].

Amount Spent

Amount of money spent by the consumers on street food per day varied from person to person. The majority of consumers in Calcutta spent Rs. 40–400 per month on street foods, while 1–2% spent as high as Rs. 700 and 1,000 per month. On average, regular consumers spent Rs. 250 per month [18]. In Hyderabad, it ranged from Rs. 30 to 150 per month [30]. Khan [59] reported that the amount of money spent by the children in Parbhani on street food was as low as Rs. 10–30 per month.

Selection of Food

Selection of the street foods by the consumers varied from person to person. In the Philippines and India the taste of the food was the primary reason for selection. Generally, the next most popular reasons for selecting street foods were their convenience/availability but never for their nutritional value [23]. Chakravarty [32] reported that in Calcutta (India) the vendors were patronized by a specific clientele not on account of cost of foods only but also due to easy accessibility, taste and variety. In Hyderabad, the majority of the consumers preferred street foods because of the variety (30%), taste (18%), convenience and low cost (12.4%) [30]. Khan [59] reported that street foods in Parbhani were preferred by the consumers on the basis of color, taste and cost. In Pune, street foods were selected by the consumers merely on the merit of taste and satiety value [26]. Consumers in Secunderabad preferred street foods to satisfy their taste and hunger [25].

The consumers in Korea considered convenience the key factor for patronizing street food vendors [7]. In a Philippino study, nutrition and value of the food came in third after taste and low cost [23].

Profile of Street Foods in Asian Countries

Variety

Given the plethora of street foods in Asian countries (table 6), there is a variety ranging from 3 to >245 breaking the monotony of daily diets. The different types of food include snack preparation, sweetmeats, beverages (alcohol, nonalcoholic, traditional) to full-course meals. Traditional foods which require lots of time and manpower for their preparation are also sold by the street vendors.

Street Foods on Special Occasions

Street food vendors beside functioning during normal days also sell food to meet the public demands on special occasions like festivals, public meetings, fairs, or any other events when a large number of people congregate on an ad hoc basis to do profitable business [60, 61].

Table 6. Variety of street foods sold in Asia

Country	Varieties
Bangladesh	128
China	31
India	100
Indonesia	>245
Israel	5
Japan	9
Korea	4
Malaysia	55
Nepal	35
Pakistan	5
Philippines	220
Thailand (Bangkok)	217
Vietnam	3

In India, traditionally street foods were sold mostly both in rural as well as in the urban areas during festive occasions, public meetings, fairs, sport events, and state functions such as independence day and republic day [50]. The number of vendors increased during the festive occasion when compared to a normal day [44]. Unlike in Bangladesh it has been observed that during the holy month of Ramadan (Islamic month of fasting), the number of vendors fell by 45% [28]. Special type of foods were sold on the festive occasions in the twin cities of Hyderabad and Secunderabad [43, 44, 48, 62].

Selling of street foods on holidays and during religious festivals is common in Malaysia [3]. There was an increase in the amount and variety of these foods when compared to normal days. The most important celebrations were Hariraya Puasa, following the fasting month of Ramadan of Muslims, the Chinese New Year and the Indian Deepavali. Joshi [2] reported that street foods were sold near temples and places where ceremonies and the festivals were organized in Nepal. Similar observations were also made in Bangladesh [9].

Seasonality
Different types of street food were sold in different seasons in the twin cities of Hyderabad (India) [44]. Beverages like sugar cane juice, coconut water, fresh fruit juice, synthetic juice, buttermilk, soda, lassi, faluda, kulfi, ice cream, and ice bars were sold during the summer season. Snack items like bajji (mirchi, onion), halem, were more common in the winter seasons, and corn cobs, bajji, in the rainy seasons. Battcock [9] reported that in Bangladesh different street foods are sold in village markets at different times of the year.

Table 7. Types of processing methods used in the preparation of street food in Asian countries

Country	Processing methods	Year	Ref. No.
China	deep frying, stir frying, steaming, boiling, roasting, marinating, salad tossing, in cold serving	1993	49
India	roasting in sand/flame/fire/griddle, grilling, boiling, simmering, steaming, pressure cooking, mincing, marinating, soaking, germinating, wet grinding, fermentation, cooking, cooking on plate on slow heat, shallow frying, deep frying, popping, baking, freezing, drying	1986, 1994	26, 63
Malaysia (Penang)	boiling, frying, sautering, grilling, griddling, fermentation	1990	3
Pakistan	cooking, frying, soaking, grinding, fermenting, roasting, filtering, freezing	1992	66
Thailand	steaming, boiling, fermentation, grinding, roasting, frying, smoking	1994	27

In the 'Boishakh' month (April 15 to May 15) green 'mango achar' (pickle) is made while in the 'Zoistho' month (May 15 to June 15) 'am shokto' (mango leather) is made. There was an increase in the number of vendors in the summer months in India [63]. Rural folk who do not find work during the dry summer in villages, flock to cities to do brisk sales of urban street foods and once the rainy season sets they go back to their fields for agricultural work. Similar observations were made in other Asian countries also. For example, in Chonburi (Thailand) 1,370 vendors were present in the dry season, while their number was reduced to 948 in the rainy season [28]. In Bogor, the total number of vendors dropped only by 5% in the prime agricultural season. Perdigon [3] reported that in Penang, the peak seasons of street food vending were the summer and festival time.

Type of Fuel Used

Type of fuel used by the street food vendors as source of energy for the preparation of street food varies from country to country in Asia. In a few parts of India, the street food vendors used kerosene and hard coke as a source of energy for cooking food [25, 26, 64]. Vendors used gas cylinders as a source of energy for cooking in Singapore [4] whereas in Pakistan and Penang (Malaysia) the majority of the vendors used charcoal and gas as a source of

Table 8. Type of containers used for storage, serving and packaging street foods in Asian countries

City/country	Storage/display containers	Serving containers	Packaging materials	Ref. No.
India				
Hyderabad and Secunderabad	wooden containers/ compartments, metal bins, vessels, glass jars, bottles, plastic containers, porcelain jars, clay/mud pots, jars, bowls, leaves (dried), cups/plates, folding tables	hand to hand, plates – steel, porcelain, glasses – metal-steel glass, plastic mugs – glass, porcelain, earthenware bowls, newspaper, stationary waste; leaves – fresh/dried, cups, plates (banana, adda, etc.)	tin foil, newspaper, dried/fresh leaves (banana, palas, adda), polythene bags, paper bags, cups/cones, plastic wrap	25, 30, 63, 68
Calcutta	–	tumblers – glass, steel, brass, ceramic, earthenware	–	18
Malaysia (Penang)	plastic bags	–	wrappers, platic bags, wax papers, old newspaper	3
Thailand (Bangkok)	wooden plates, bowls, metal, glass containers, earthenware, insulated boxes, plastic bags	plates – ceramic, plastic, glass tumblers/bottles	plastic bags, polystyrene foam boxes, banana leaves, bamboo baskets	27
Indonesia (West Java)	–	–	banana leaves, bamboo baskets	69

cooking fuel [3, 31, 65, 66]. Perdigon [3] also reported that very few vendors in Penang also used wood.

Hutabarat [27] reported that vendors in Bangkok (Thailand) used electricity in addition to charcoal and gas.

Processing Methods

Different types of processing methods are used by the street food vendors in the preparation of street foods in Asian countries. These include both traditional and modern methods (table 7).

Storage and Serving Containers and Packaging Materials

A variety of materials are used for making storage/serving containers and also for packaging the street foods (table 8). These vary from the traditional banana leaves, earthenware, glass, metal and recent innovations like plastic. New biodegradable packaging materials developed in countries like Japan are also used for packaging street foods [67].

Snack items like 'pani puri' was served hand to hand by some vendors. Such a unique method of serving 'pani puri' is not practiced with regard to any other foods. It is a direct method of serving which can be termed as 'hand to hand'. The vendor takes the puffed 'puri' presses it with the thumb so that a hole is made and dips it into a vessel containing masala pani, and hands it over to the customer repeating the process 8–10 times. The customer consumes the item as soon as he receives it from the vendor [63].

The prepared foods were displayed on folding tables, trays, etc., without any protective covering, exposed to dust, fumes, insects, smoke, etc. Only some of the containers are either covered with lids or merely with a piece of cloth [25, 27, 63].

Use of Leftover Items

Limited data is available on the utilization of the leftover foods by the street food vendors in the different Asian countries. The practices vary from place to place and vendor to vendor. In Secunderabad (India) the leftover food items were either thrown away (60%) or given to the poor (6%), fed to the dogs (2%), taken home and consumed (18%), or sold the next day in some modified form (5.3%); some of the vendors (8.7%) did not reveal any information regarding the usage [25]. However, the majority of the vendors in Hyderabad used the leftover food at home (54%) while the rest utilized it the next day (46%) [30]. Similar observations were also made in Pune [26], Penang (Malaysia) [3], and Nepal (Khatmandu) [7]. In Penang (Malaysia), the leftover foods were taken home by the vendor or his assistant for consumption. Leftover food was also recycled for the next day's business which would add to the revenue and increase the profit [3]. About 48% of the vendors in Khatmandu sold the unsold food the next day [7].

Water Facilities

Various studies conducted in the Asian countries have revealed several problems pertaining to the quality of street foods. Among these the most crucial problem was lack of an adequate supply of potable water for cooking, cleaning, cleaning of mixing and eating utensils, personal hygiene, for use in beverages, drinking, etc. Street food vendors in Manikgunj (Bangladesh) used water drawn from deep wells in all the major selling areas while in Pune (India) only 47% of the vendors had municipal tap water and the rest used water from other sources like a borewell, etc. [26]. Similar observations were also made in Bogor (Indonesia) [21] and Penang (Malaysia) [3]. Some of the vendors also purchased water in containers from private faucets connected to the water mains [3]. In Khatmandu (Nepal) and Pakistan (at the railway station) municipal water was available [7, 31] unlike in China and Korea where tap water facilities were nonexistent [7, 49].

Due to the unavailability of adequate water most of the vendors in Asian countries reused the same water for washing, rinsing, etc. For example, Bharathi [30] reported that vendors in Hyderabad washed the plates in unclean water; the same bucket of water was reused again and again to wash the plates. Similar observations were also made in Secunderabad, Pune (India), Korea, and the Philippines, etc. [7, 21, 63].

Disposal of Waste

Disposal of waste water and refuse including garbage was shown to be an almost universal problem in most of the Asian countries [12]. Studies conducted in China revealed that the availability of liquid and solid waste disposal facilities were often nonexistent [49]. Similarly, in Bombay (India) there was no system for garbage disposal. All leftover waste material was thrown into nearby gutters on the roadside [56]. As an exception, only 65% of the areas in Nepal used by street vendors had waste disposal containers available while the rest had none. If there are no facilities for disposal of liquid drainage, waste water and garbage, such wastes are littered in the streets encouraging the breeding of mosquitoes and flies. These pests carry and spread pathogens. Exposed raw materials and ready-to-eat foods sold in such locations are very susceptible to contamination by the flies. The linkage between house flies and diarrheal disease has been well documented in the past [58, 70]. Hawkers in Singapore are required to use plastic bags for refuse and bulk bins are provided nearby for waste disposal [71].

Place of Preparation

The place of preparation of street food in the Asian countries by vendors varied from country to country and vendor to vendor depending upon the facilities available near the vending site. In China, the street foods were mainly prepared and sold on the spot [49]. Chakravarthy [32] reported that in Calcutta (India) street foods were classified into three categories: (1) prepared at a central place for distribution (cottage industries); (2) prepared at the home of the vendor and sold on the street; (3) prepared and sold at the street food stalls. In Hyderabad, the preparation of the street food was carried out on the spot by 76% of the vendors, at home by 6%, and the rest of the vendors did the preparations both at home and on the spot depending upon the item and situation [30]. Similar observations were made in Secunderabad [25], Malaysia [13] and Khatmandu [7].

Bryan et al. [66] reported that 'Chat', a regionally popular food in Pakistan was prepared half a mile from where they vended. The way the street foods were sold by the street food vendors in Asian countries varied from place to place. For example, in Bangladesh, the street foods scenario reveals mainly four distinct features, i.e. vendors carrying their items on head or shoulder, carrying their food products in small vans, vendors operating in thatched houses or in semifurnished buildings and vendors who sit out in the open [7]. In China, there were five types such as regular buildings, simple buildings, fixed stalls, kiosks and mobile vendors [49]. Similarly, in India, there were permanent buildings, semipermanent wooden stalls, wooden movable carts, bamboo baskets, freezing chambers, tables in the open air, and persons carrying on head or shoulder [26, 63]. In Indonesia, vendors carry their wares by hand on shoulders, poles or by use of wheeled transport such as bicycles or pushcarts [72]. The vendors in Laos sold on mobile trolleys and on tables in the open [7]. In Malaysia, the street food vendors were vending the foods through mobile stalls, motor vehicles, bicycles, tricycles, and fixed kiosks [7, 13]. In Pakistan, vendors used permanent stands, stalls and carts [66]. In the Philippines, the street vendors mostly used tricycles [21]. Street foods such as snacks were sold by cycle trailer mobile shops in Suriyawewa (Sri Lanka) [73]. In Bangkok (Thailand), vendors used to sell their wares by carrying them on shoulder poles, by wheeled transport, stalls, booths, tents and kiosks [27].

There are mainly two types of vending vehicles, i.e. mobile (ambulatory) and stationary (stay put), used by street food vendors in the Asian countries. The number varied from place to place and country to country. In Bangladesh, there were mostly mobile pushcarts which were usually the province of men and were positioned at the same intersection every day [21]. In China, the vending vehicles were mostly stationary (60%), while 39.3% were mobile stalls [40]. Seth and Bhat [74] and Bhat et al. [63] reported that most of the vending stalls were stationary in the twin cities of Hyderabad and Secunderabad (India) while the rest were mobile units. In contrast, in Indonesia, Laos, Malaysia, the Philippines and Sri Lanka, most of the stalls were mobile [3, 7, 72]. In Pakistan and Bangladesh, both types of vending vehicles were common [27, 31, 65, 66].

Materials used in the construction of vending vehicles in Asia vary from country to country. Prakash [50] reported that the vending vehicles in India were made of wood. They consist of a wooden board platform mounted at a height on a chassis of four bicycle wheels held together by steel rods and strip framing (primary structure). Similar findings were also reported by Bhat et al. [63]. In Pakistan, the vendors' stand was constructed of wood and glass at the upper half both at the front and sides [66]. It was painted and lettered in bright colors. A newly designed pushcart was prepared by Wirakartakusumah [72] in Indonesia. The pushcart was constructed using an iron steel and aluminum frame and fiberglass for the body, stainless steel was used in the preparation area.

Location of Vending Vehicles
Street foods have become very popular in the Asian countries for various reasons and are available at the places where required, i.e. around factories,

offices, schools, universities, transit points, marketplaces [12, 58, 75]: in Bangladesh [21], Yinchang and Pugu city of China [76], India [25, 50, 63, 64, 68], Indonesia [21], Malaysia [7], Laos [7], the Philippines [21], Pakistan [31] and Thailand [27].

In most of the Asian countries, for example, Bangladesh, Thailand, the Philippines and Indonesia, the truly mobile vendor is in the minority. Most carts are pushed to the same location each day and removed at night. Some vendors have regular positions, for example, schools and cinemas. Even women selling from baskets carried on their heads tend to squat in the same place every day, such as next to the bus station or outside the marketplace. There are some really mobile vendors using bicycles selling bread or ices or shoulder balance poles allowing a tiny stool to be carried on one end to balance the sweets or tea on the other. Such vendors follow a regular route every day. These mobile vendors accounted for 18% in Chonburi (Thailand) [28].

About 80% of the street food trade in Iloilo (Philippines) and Bogor (Indonesia) is concentrated in residential areas, rather than the central city area. In the smaller towns, distances are not so great and the vendors are more spatially dispersed. There are many 'doorstep' vendors – predominantly women who set up a table and chairs on the sidewalk outside their homes [15].

Quality of Street Foods in Asia

Physical Quality

Studies conducted in Asia involved the analysis of foods for their nutritional quality, presence of food additives and contaminants and microbial quality. In tropical countries, the street foods are always exposed to dust, vehicle fumes, flies, insects, etc. [25, 26, 30, 64, 68, 76]. However, precautions are taken by very few vendors. For example, Bharathi [30] reported that in Hyderabad (India) only 18% of the vendors were using protective covering like glass doors (for pushcarts) or glass cases to cover the street foods. Similar observations were also made in Pune and Secunderabad (India). Around 32% of the vendors used glass covers to protect the street foods [26] in Secunderabad and only 28% of the vendors had a few items covered. Besides, the pushcarts were located adjacent to public urinals and near garbage dumps (64%) [25].

A study conducted in Calcutta (India) revealed that no excessive amounts of filth, dirt or dust were observed in the quantitative analysis of street food samples. The samples were also found satisfactory from the point of view of appearance, smell, taste, edibility and freshness [32]. The quality of street foods in Dhaka (Bangladesh), Korea and Thailand, in general were below acceptable standards. Statistical data in Vietnam from 1980 to 1990 showed that about 50% of street food samples did not meet the hygienic requirements [7].

Chemical Quality

The different aspects of chemical quality of street foods in different Asian countries which were studied included food additives, toxins, and heavy metals. Several studies have shown that a number of banned food additives were being used by the street vendors in different food preparations [6]. Presence of banned coloring like metanil yellow, orange II in popular sweetmeats such as 'jelebi' and 'bundi laddu' and rhodamine B, auromine orange G in sugar candy were detected in India. Other sweetmeat samples like cotton candy, floss candy, coconut burfi samples in India also showed the presence of banned coloring like rhodamine B and orange G [24, 26, 34, 43, 57].

Stoots et al. [77] reported that non-food-grade additives such as textile coloring agents were detected in several street food samples in West Java (Indonesia). The study also confirmed the use of banned coal tar colors in soft drinks and other foods [6, 23]. Kim et al. [78] reported that 36% of the soft drink samples prepared and sold by local street vendors in Hanoi (Vietnam) showed the presence of banned colors. Of the 74 samples collected in 5 districts of Bangkok (Thailand), all contained acceptable levels of permitted coloring agents [79].

Several studies conducted in the Asian countries have revealed the presence of heavy metals in the food samples sold by the street vendors. For example, in Pune (India) metallic contaminants were within the permissible limits in some of the street foods. Snack food such as alutar, bajji, onion bajji, masala dosa and dahi vada showed higher values for copper, i.e. more than 1.5 ppm (6.86–22.36 ppm) [26]. The Indonesian study also confirmed the presence of heavy metals like lead and iron in samples of hot dogs, bakmi/bihun bakso (a wheat/rice noodle soup with meat balls) and nasi uduk, steamed rice with coconut milk and spices. The contamination resulted from atmospheric pollution, i.e. specially from automobile exhaust fumes [6, 23]. Similar observations were also made by Joshi [2] in Khatmandu (Nepal). He reported that lead was found in most of the sweets sold by street vendors near the bus parks. Hutabarat [27] also revealed the presence of lead in different street food samples such as meals (trace to 3.04 ppm), beverages (trace to 1.05 ppm) and snacks (0.27–4.32 ppm) sold by the street food vendors in Bangkok (Thailand).

Seth [25] and Waghray and Bhat [43] revealed the presence of *Lathyrus sativus* (a harmful pulse) in some of the street food samples such as mirchi bajji, vada and bonda, sold by vendors in the twin cities of Hyderabad and Secunderabad (India). In contrast, in the samples analyzed in Calcutta, *L. sativus* was not detected [32, 62].

Some of the street food samples sold by the vendors in Asian countries also revealed the presence of mycotoxin such as aflatoxin. Winnarno and Allain [16] reported that 17% of street foods containing peanuts sold by vendors in Indonesia were contaminated with aflatoxin at levels above 30 ppb. Joshi [2] in Khatmandu (Nepal) reported that 35% of the samples collected from street vendors were contaminated with aflatoxin, of which 25% were heavily contaminated. Hutabarat [27] revealed the presence of alfatoxins within permissible levels (20 ppb) in street meal samples collected from street vendors in Bangkok. In another study, Vatanasuchart [79] reported that of 74 samples of Thai foods collected from 5 districts of Bangkok (Thailand) one sample of Somtom was contaminated with aflatoxin at 0.96 µg/kg. Unlike the samples collected from the street food vendors in metro Manilla [80] and Calcutta [32] which were negative for aflatoxin.

Very meager information is available pertaining to the pesticide residues in the street food samples sold by the vendors in Asian countries. Joshi [2] reported the occurrence of pesticide residues in green vegetables and other food products sold by the street vendors in Khatmandu (Nepal). In Sri Lanka pesticide residues were also found in fresh fruits and vegetables sold by street food vendors [6, 23]. Presence of pesticide residues like tetradifon and dicofol was observed in 5.6% of street meal samples and 16% of beverage samples collected from the street food vendors in Bangkok (Thailand) [27]. Another study conducted by Vatanasuchart [79] revealed the presence of tetradefon (<0.01 mg/kg) in two samples of orange juice.

Several preservatives are used by street food vendors in different Asian countries. Lianghui et al. [81] reported that street food vendors in Shandong province of China misused the chemical preservative – sodium nitrite. The presence of mold inhibitors like sodium benzoate and sodium metabisulphite in street foods was detected in Indonesia. Other types of texture modifiers such as 'bleng', a borate-containing salt, were found in noodles, tapioca and chips [6]. Many vendors also used monosodium glutamate, a flavor enhancer, in their foods. A sample of baso (meat balls) was found to contain no protein. It was presumed that instead of meat, beef fat and monosodium glutamate had been used [23]. Perdigon [3] reported the presence of an illegal preservative (boric acid) used by street food vendors in Malaysia to bleach and give shine to the food product such as looseefun (rice noodles). In Sri Lanka, formalin was detected as a substitute for ice in preserving fish sold by the street food vendors [23]. Hutabarat [27] revealed the presence of the preservative sodium benzoate in excess of permitted levels in beverages sold by the street food vendors in Bangkok (Thailand). In another study conducted by Vatanasuchart [79] benzoic acid was detected in 10 beverage and 2 snack samples in the range of 51.9–347.4 and 61.6–192.5 mg/kg, respectively, from the 74 food samples (meals, beverages and snacks) collected from street vendors in 5 districts of Bangkok (Thailand).

Very few studies have been conducted in the Asian countries pertaining to the use of artificial sweeteners. Saccharin was detected in nonalcoholic beverages like sarbats and tea sold by the street food vendors in Pune (India) [6, 26]. Another study conducted in Pune by Gandham [82] also revealed the presence of artificial sweeteners like saccharin in 4/46 solid samples like sweet confectioneries, bakery products and 50% (17/34) of the liquid food samples such as sherbets, ice balls and ice creams. Kim et al. [78] also observed the presence of artificial sweeteners like saccharin, cyclamate and dulcine in place of sugar in soft drinks (25%) prepared and sold by local vendors in Hanoi (Vietnam). In contrast, only 1 of the 74 street food samples of beverages snacks and meals collected from 5 districts of Bangkok (Thailand) revealed the presence of artificial sweeteners [79].

Very meager information is available on the usage of reheated/reused oil by the street food vendors and the presence of adulterants in the cooking oil used by them in the Asian countries. Many street food vendors in Coimbatore and Hyderabad (India) prepared the food in reheated oil [30, 83]. Hema et al. [57] observed the presence of mineral oil and castor oil in the edible oil which was used by the street food vendors in Coimbatore. The cooking oil used by the vendors in Secunderabad and Calcutta (India) indicated the presence of argemone oil which contains toxic alkaloids [25, 32].

Nutritional Quality

Nutritional investigations carried out in many Asian countries revealed that freshly cooked traditional street foods are a source of various nutrients. It is believed that many low income families would be worse off if there were no street foods [56]. According to Chakravarthy [32] and Chakravarthy and Canet [18], 15 street food samples were analyzed in Calcutta (India) for their protein, fat and carbohydrate energy values. Street foods were nutritionally well balanced and provided approximately 200 kcal energy per food worth of Rs. 1 (USD = 35 Indian rupees). The protein and calorie content of the street food content of the street food samples old in the twin cities of Hyderabad and Secunderabad (India), ranged from 6.4 to 8.3% and 303 to 390 kcal/100 g (gold fingers); 8.3–9.3% and 325–359 kcal/100 g (Muruku); 19.0–20.4 and 259–304 kcal/100 g (roasted peas), respectively [53]. In Parbhani, protein content of the various snack foods ranged between 0.01 and 24.3/100 g; fat 0–42.8 g/100 g; energy 7–589 kcal; calcium 8–208 mg/100 g; iron 0.03–2.5 mg/

100 g. Among the different snack preparations, the nutritional quality of 'Kharmure' was the best as it provided the highest quantities of protein (24.3 g), fat (42.8 g), energy (589 kcal), and iron (2.5 mg/100 g sample) [59]. Another study conducted in Parbhani (India) revealed that the protein digestibility of different snack foods sold by the vendors near slum areas ranged from 11.2 to 54.6%, protein content 3.0 to 17.9 g, fat 0.1 to 37.18 g/100 g sample; minerals: iron 0.19 to 7.44 mg and copper, zinc and manganese ranged from 0.02 to 0.93 mg/100 g sample [33].

Studies conducted in Pune for nutrient content of street food meals showed that the higher the moisture content, the lower the nutritional value of that particular food. Fat content was maximum in fried foods. Deep-fried foods showed appreciable amounts of fat content and foods that were shallow fried had comparatively lower fat content ranging from 5.3 to 17.00%. The calorie content varied from 95.4 to 380.87 kcal. Protein-rich foods were mostly non-vegetarian dishes. The protein content varied from 31.5 to 24%. Protein value in several preparations was enhanced due to the presence of groundnuts in the recipe and most of the snacks were prepared from pulse flour which enriched the protein content. The value ranged from 0.62 to 17.1%. The caloric value of the snacks was quite high 72.9 to 488 kcal compared to cost. The samples of ice cream and kulfi, a frozen dessert consisting of khoa, sugar and cardamon, were nutritionally sound and their caloric values were appreciable (62.0–197.93 kcal). However, they were not found to be a cheap source of refreshment [26].

A number of fresh fruit samples were found to be the richest sources of essential vitamins, mineral content and fiber. The food energy and protein value of cooked street food is certainly higher than that which could be obtained from prepackaged processed foods at the going marketplace [26]. Studies conducted in Indonesia revealed that average energy content of street foods ranges from 5 to 679 cal per 100 g.

Hutabarat [27] reported that the nutritional value of the different street meals varied depending upon their type of composition in Bangkok. For street meals analyzed, the average calorie content ranged between 37 and 204 cal, average protein between 1.6 and 19.74%, average fat between 0.64 and 11.9%, average fiber between 0.30 and 1.9%, average carbohydrate between 1.5 and 24.5% and average sugar content between 2.1 and 23.3%. The average energy values for the snack preparations ranged between 46 to 365 cal, protein content between 0.09 and 15.6%, fat content between 0.32 and 30.5%, fiber content between 0.28 and 3.00%, carbohydrate content 6.9 and 65% and sugar content between 6.3 and 58.2%. Though calories of individual street foods are low, since they are eaten in combination of two to four different dishes at a time, the overall nutritional value was considered good.

Studies were conducted by Nagalakshmi [84] on the energy, vitamin C and sugar content of beverages sold by the street food vendors in Hyderabad and were found to be adequate. Very few studies have been conducted relating to the cost of street foods and its nutrient content. For example, studies conducted in Calcutta (India) revealed that street food provided nearly 1,000 cal from an average of Rs. 5 to 6 only in 1994, 1 USD equalled Rs. 33) [32]. Jadhav [33] reported that in Parbhani (India) Kharmure provided 18 g/100 g of protein for Rs. 3 and bread at the same cost provided more proteins, trace minerals, energy and satiety. More than half of the RDA of protein, vitamin C, vitamin A and iron could be got from a Rp 300 rice-based meal in Bogor (Indonesia) [15].

Microbial Quality

Several studies have been conducted on the microbial quality of different snack preparations sold by the street food vendors in various Asian countries. For example, Chakravarthy [32] and Chakravarthy et al. [33] reported that the microbial quality of the snack foods sold by the street food vendors in Calcutta was not satisfactory. Detailed analysis of the food samples showed that the standard plate counts of fermented products like dahi vada and idli, was high as compared to other varieties of samples. Among the fermented products, idli (254×10/g), dahivada (420×10/g) had higher counts than dosa (37.3×10/g), presumably due to the heat treatment (frying) during its preparation. But few unfermented ones, e.g. ghungi (188.8×10/g) and alu kabli (33.4×10/g), also indicated high SP counts and some also contained pathogenic organisms. *Escherichia coli* was detected in 55% of the samples. The presence of coagulase *Staphylococcus aureus* was noted in 7 of 52 samples. All the samples of Fuchka indicated the presence of pathogenic organisms. Almost all the snack samples showed the presence of yeast and mold in minute quantities [33].

Kaul and Aggarwal [85] examined the microbial load of common chat (popular snack) products like paprichat, bhallachat, behlpuri and fruit chat sold by the various vendors and shop owners in Chandigarh. The total and specific microbial counts ranged from 10^8 to 10^{10} cfu/g and 10^3 to 10^7 cfu/g, respectively. An increase in microbial count by 1 to 3 log cycles was seen after storage for 16 and 24 h at room temperature. Hema et al. [57] also studied the microbial quality of 8 commonly consumed street foods including raw foods, fried items, hot and cold foods, and sweets. They reported that all food samples had high microbial counts ($> 100,000$ cfu/g). Similar studies were also conducted by Bharathi [30] on the 10 most popular foods sold on the streets of Hyderabad. The samples showed the presence of coliform bacteria, *E. coli* and fungal growth. Among the street foods panipuri, samosa, cutlets, ragada, were found to be highly contaminated by fungal organisms (0.07×10^3

to 0.4×10^3). In addition, bhelpuri, egg bonda, masala vada, alu bonda, mirchi and alu bajji were also contaminated by fungal organisms at a moderate to lower rate (0.03×10^2 to 0.09×10^2). All the street foods examined were found to be contaminated with *E. coli*. Studies conducted on the microbial quality of 30 popular snack preparations sold by street vendors in Pune revealed that among all the snacks items, bhalpuri had high microbial counts compared to panipuri and ragada pattis. Unlike samples of snack items like uttappa, upma, shira, bread masala, sabudana khichri and omelette which were served hot on demand were free of microbial contamination [26]. Microbiological studies conducted on the food samples collected from street vendors in Bogor (Indonesia) also showed the presence of *Salmonella* species [6].

Bryan et al. [66] studied the microbial quality of chat and its items displayed by the street vendors in Pakistan. They reported that among the food samples taken all but one had mesophillic aerobic colony counts that exceeded one million cfu/g, while eight had counts greater than 10^8. Coliforms were present in all of the 18 samples and all but one exceeded 10^4; eight of the samples exceeded 10^6. *Bacillus cereus* was isolated from 5 of 16 samples. *Clostridium perfringens* was not isolated from 12 samples. Upwards to 5.6×10^5 *S. aureus* per gram was isolated from 8 of 14 samples. Staphylococcal enterotoxin type A was produced by isolates from potatoes after peeling, cutting and stacking on trays.

Beverages

Many studies have been conducted on the microbial quality of various types of beverages sold by the street food vendors in different Asian countries. Chakravarthy [32] and Chakravarthy et al. [62] reported that the beverage samples (both milk based and other) collected from the street food vendors in Calcutta (India) were not satisfactory for their microbial quality. Detailed analysis of milk-based beverages like lassi showed the presence of coliforms (6.20/g), *E. coli* (3.40/g), yeast (12.10×10/g), mold (4.2×10/g), *Salmonella* species and high standard plate counts (564.80×10/g). Similar results were also reported from Madras and Pune. Pillai et al. [86] reported that the total viable counts and aerobic spore counts (3.86×10^7 cfu/g; 3.26×10^5 cfu/g) were higher in the lassi samples collected from local vendors in Madras when compared to those from private manufacturers and organized dairies in Madras city (India). Studies conducted in Pune on the microbial quality of lassi also revealed the presence of coliforms and fecal coliforms $\geq 180/100$ ml in 60 and 40% of the samples [26].

Bryan et al. [66] reported that the lassi sold by the street vendors in Pakistan showed the presence of coliforms (4.4×10^5 g/ml), mesophillic aerobic colony counts or aerobic plate counts (6.6×10^7 g/ml), and *S. aureus* ($<10^2$ g/ml).

Another study conducted on the microbial quality of lassi sold by the street vendors at a bus station in Pakistan also showed the presence of mesophilic aerobic colony count or aerobic plate count ($<10^2$ g/ml), and *B. cereus* ($<10^2$ g/ml) [31].

Bryan et al. [65] also studied the microbial quality of beverages (like banana milk shake, etc.) sold by the vendors in a mountain resort town in Pakistan. The results revealed the presence of mesophillic aerobic colony counts or aerobic plate counts 1.4×10^6 g/ml to 1.4×10^8 g/ml, coliforms $<10^2$ to 2×10^5 g/ml, *S. aureus* $<10^2$ g/ml, and *B. cereus* $<10^2$ g/ml. Milk also showed the presence of *Salmonella*.

Nagalakshmi [84] reported that the fruit juices like sugar cane juice, pineapple juice and lime juice sold by the street food vendors in Hyderabad (India) were of poor microbial quality. The standard plate count for sugar cane juice ranges from 24.0×10^5 to 36.5^5 per ml of juice, for pineapple juice ranges from 1.13×10^5 to 30.4×10^5 per ml of juice, for lime juice ranges from 0.03×10^5 to 11.8×10^5 per ml. The yeast and mold count for sugar cane juice ranges from 36×10^4 to 81.7×10^4 per ml of juice, for pineapple juice (1.87×10^4 to 21.0×10^4 per ml) and for lime (0.01×10^4 to 1.43×10^4 per ml). Each counts for the sugar cane and pineapple juices were 0.63×10^4 to 8.35×10^4 per ml of juice; 3.75×10^4 to 117.5×10^4 per ml of juice, respectively, while lime juice did not show the presence of *E. coli*. Similar studies were also conducted in Pune on the microbial quality of different beverages like sugar cane juice, sherbet and fruit juice sold by street vendors. The highest contamination was found in sugar cane juice when compared with sherbet and fruit juice. All the beverages revealed the presence of coliforms and fecal coliforms and the counts were > 180/ml (96 and 24% of sugar cane juice, 69.3 and 34.9% sherbets, 40 and 20% of fruit juices). Sherbets and fruit juice samples also contained *E. coli* (6.1 and 20%) and 20% of the fruit juice samples also showed the presence of enteropathogenic *E. coli* [26]. The Escedol samples (a beverage consisting of sago dough lumps (cendol) mixed with coconut milk and sugar syrup, and added shredded ice) collected from the street food vendors in West Java (Indonesia) were highly contaminated with bacteria (APC > 10 million cfu/g, EC $> 100,000$ cfu/g, LABC > 1 million cfu/g) [69].

Bryan et al. [31] also studied the microbial quality of beverages like sugar cane juice, sherbet sandal, etc., sold by the street vendors near a bus station in Pakistan. The results revealed the presence of mesophillic aerobic colony counts or aerobic plate count (1.6×10^4 to 1×10^6 g/ml), coliforms (2×10^3 to 9.8×10^5 g/ml).

The beverages sold in the different locations of Bangkok (Thailand) were of poor microbial quality. Soft drink samples (n$=$66) had high total viable counts (less than 10–8 cfu/ml) and high levels of *E. coli* and also showed the presence of *C. perfringens* and *S. aureus* (3.7, 18.0%), respectively [87].

Hutabarat [27] reported that the beverages sold by the street food vendors in Bangkok showed the presence of Coliform bacteria, *E. coli*, yeast and mold. The values ranged between 0 and 10^8 cfu/ml (total plate count), $0 > 2,400$ MPN/ml (coliform bacteria), 0–2,400 MPN/100 ml (*E. coli*), $0–10^6$ cfu/ml (yeast) and $0–10^3$ cfu/ml (mold). Statistical analysis revealed that neither the location of selling, the selling periods nor the particular beverage itself had any significant effect on the microbial quality of the beverages.

Coliform bacteria in beverages were indicative of improper hygienic practices. Fecal contamination came from vendors and utensils or it may also have come from some ingredients including nonpotable water ice. Coliform bacteria in beverages may have come from the water and ice used in their preparation. This conclusion was supported by the laboratory research for drinking water and ice for human consumption.

Beverage samples also showed the presence of *C. perfringens* (0–17%) and *S. aureus* (0–50%). There was no significant difference based on the locations of selling for contamination with *C. perfringens* though there was *S. aureus*. The samples collected from the transportation areas had highest incidence of *S. aureus* contamination at 37.55% while 13.4% of samples collected from the university and 6.7% from marketplaces were contaminated. Only 15.3% of the samples collected from housing areas were contaminated by *C. perfringens*.

Very meager information is available on the microbial quality of traditional beverages like neera, ice used in the beverages, and masala pani in the Asian countries. Neera (naturally secreted sap of palm tree) showed the presence of coliform counts more than 180/100 ml in 20% of the samples and fecal coliforms were also more than 180/100 ml in 10% of the samples collected from the street vendors in Pune (India) [26].

Ice used by the street vendors in preparation of sugar cane juice in Hyderabad (India) was of poor microbial quality. It showed the presence of *E. coli* (1.05×10^3/ml), plate counts (2.32×10^5/ml) and yeast and mold count 3.45×10^4/ml [84]. About 80% of the ice samples collected from the street food vendors in Pune (India) also showed the presence of coliform count more than 180/100 ml and 10% of the samples also contained fecal coliforms more than 180/100 ml. The presence of enteropathogenic *E. coli* from 10% of the ice samples examined indicated gross contamination of fecal origin [26]. Of the 16 samples of water and ice cubes collected from street vendors in Khatmandu (Nepal), only 1 sample showed the presence of *E. coli*, fecal *Streptococci* and *Salmonella* species [2]. Hutabarat [27] reported that 100% of the ice samples collected from street vendors in Bangkok (Thailand) contained coliform bacteria and 80% of the ice samples also showed the presence of *E. coli* while 20% of the ice samples showed the presence of *C. perfringens.*

The microbial quality of masala pani (water with spices) used by the 'panipuri' vendors in the streets of Pune (India) was of poor quality. Of the 14 masala pani samples collected, 10 (71.4%) were positive for coliform bacteria while 7 (60%) were positive for fecal coliforms. Enteropathogenic *E. coli* was isolated from 3 (21.4%) samples and *S. newport* was isolated from one pani sample (7.1%) [26].

Cut Vegetables and Fruits

Studies have also been conducted in the Asian countries pertaining to the microbial quality of cut fruits sold by the street vendors. For example, Guha et al. [88] studied the bacterial quality of cucumber slices sold by the vendors in Calcutta (India). The results revealed that the average standard plate counts of psychrophillic and lipolylic bacteria, mold, enterococci, coliform and fecal coliform were 43.8×10^3, 5.4×10^3, 2.3×10^3, 1.8×10^3, 0.8×10^3, 1.3×10^3, 2.9 and 0.5 per gram of sample, respectively. Coliform, fecal coliform and enterococci were detected in 94.2, 77.6 and 89.7% of the samples, respectively. In 19 samples, the presence of *E. coli* was observed. A small number of coagulase-positive *S. aureus* was also detected in a few samples, while other pathogenic forms like *Salmonella, Shigella, Vibrio cholerae* and *V. parahaemo-lyticus* were not detected. The microbial quality of different kinds of cut fruits sold by the vendors in Pune was also studied. Cut fruits like watermelon, pineapple, and jack fruit showed high coliform counts indicating unhygienic handling of these fruits. 60% of the watermelons had higher coliform counts (4.8×10^3/g) as street food sellers always sell this fruit cut in small pieces during the summer.

Water

Very vague reports pertaining to the microbial quality of water used by the street food vendors in the Asian countries are available. Chakravarthy [32] and Chakravarthy et al. [62] conducted the microbiological examination of water which was used by the street food vendors for washing, drinking in four selected survey areas in Calcutta (India). The results revealed that the water was found to be nonpotable in nature due to the presence of coliform and fecal coliforms in most of the samples. Similar results were also observed by Nagalakshmi [84] who studied the microbial quality of water used by the street vendors of Hyderabad in the preparation of sugar cane juice. The standard plate count were 1.72×10^5/ml) yeast and mold count 1.24×10^4/ml and *E. coli* (0.85×10^3/ml). In another study, 219 water samples were collected from storage tanks of street food vendors at different localities in Pune (India). The results revealed that 29.6% of these water samples were not confirming the standards of potability given by the WHO for drinking water. In 29.6% of the water samples coliform counts were more than 16/100 ml while fecal coliform counts were more than 16/100 ml in 15.5% of water samples, 4.5% of samples were positive for *E. coli* and 2.7% for enteropathogenic *E. coli*, *S. newport* (6,8:eh:1,2) was isolated from one stored water sample collected from a 'panipuri' vendor [26]. Joshi [2] reported that 1 of 16 samples of water and ice collected from the street vendors in Khatmandu (Nepal) showed the presence of *E. coli*, fecal *Streptococci* and *Salmonella* species. In another study, of 3 water samples 1 showed the presence of coliforms more than 2,400/g. *S. aureus* and *Salmonella* were also present in one sample.

Bryan et al. [31] studied the microbial quality of water and ice water which was used by the street vendors near a railway and a bus station in Pakistan. The results revealed the presence of coliforms ($<10^2$ to 10^2 g/ml); mesophilic aerobic colony counts or aerobic plate counts ($<10^2$ to 1.8×10^3 g/ml). About 80% of the water samples collected from the street food vendors in Bangkok (Thailand) were of poor microbial quality and contained coliform bacteria. While 20% of samples also contained *E. coli*, *S. aureus* was found in 10% of the drinking water (nam plau) samples and 10% of the water samples also showed the presence of mold (10^3 to 10^5 cfu/ml).

Meals

Several studies conducted in the Asian countries revealed that microbial quality of the meals sold by the street food vendors was of poor microbial quality. Liang and Yuan [76] reported that of 16 kinds of street-vended foods in Yichang city and Puqu city (China), the bacterial contamination of hot dry noodles and meats stewed in soy sauce were most serious in which total viable counts were 66.7 and 70% over 1.0×10^5/g, respectively; coliforms MPN were 71 and 81.5% over 2.4×10^4/100 g. Microbial quality of the 15 most popular meal side dishes sold by street vendors in Pune city (India) revealed that among the different foods analyzed cooked plain rice was highly contaminated with an average standard plate count of 1.79×10^7/g followed by mutton masala and mutton biryani ($1.01-1.5 \times 10^7$/g). Bajji samples were of poorest microbial quality pertaining to unhygienic conditions as it contained *E. coli* and an average of 3×10^3/g fecal coliforms [26]. Hartog et al. [69] studied the microbial quality of Nasi rames (a mixed rice dish) and Gado-Gado (steamed or cooked vegetables, tofu egg chilli and peanut sauces) sold by the street vendors in West Java (Indonesia). They reported that in general this rice dish appeared to be of acceptable microbial quality. Unlike the samples of Gado-Gado which contained high numbers of viable bacteria

(APC > 1 million cfu/g; EC > 1,000 cfu/g) and which during the vending process further increased.

Aziz [13] reported that microbial contamination of hawkers' food is a good indicator of unsanitary practices in the preparation and storage of foods. The findings on the microbial states of cooked ready-to-eat foods by the food quality control laboratory in Selangor (Malaysia) showed that from January through May 1990, foods which had lots of post-cooking and handling had total plate counts of more than 10^5 organisms/g, while fried foods, breads and flour confectionery had microbial counts of not more than 50 organisms/g. Results of the microbial analysis of the foods sold by the street vendors in Khatmandu (Nepal) indicated very high total mesophilic counts [7]. Some samples also showed the presence of *Staphylococcus* and *Salmonella* species. Bryan et al. [65] studied the microbial quality of foods such as pulse pattis and chicken sold by the street vendors in a mountain resort town in Pakistan. Coliform bacteria were isolated from 3 of 5 samples. *C. perfringens* were isolated from 2 of 7 pulse pattis, and *Salmonella* was isolated from the egg shell and chicken samples. Microbial analyses of 25 samples of foods like rice, chicken, burger, stew, etc., collected from the street ventors at a railway station in Pakistan revealed the presence of *C. perfringens* in 9 of 21 (43%) samples, four of these samples contained over 10^5 cfu/g and two contained more than 10^6. Four of 15 (27%) samples were positive for *B. cereus* and plate counts were higher ranging from $< 10^2$ to 22×10^8 cfu/g and coliforms $< 10^2$/g were present in 5 of 25 samples [31]. Similarly microbial analysis of 25 samples of foods like pulse pattis, beef, rice, and meat stew collected from the street vendors at a bus station was also poor.

Boonyaratarakornkit et al. [87] reported that street food meals sold by different vendors in Bangkok (Thailand) were of poor microbial quality. Results revealed that most of the partially cooked foods had high total viable counts and high levels of *E. coli* (MPN/g greater than 1,100). In the partially and well-cooked foods analyzed, *C. perfringens* and *S. aureus* were detected. Similar results were observed in another study conducted by Hutabarat [27] on microbial quality of the meals sold by street food vendors in Bangkok. It was also observed that 35% of the samples collected from residential areas, 64% from university areas, 29% from marketplaces, 41% from transportation areas, and 44.5% from recreation areas had a total plate count ranging from 10^6 to 10^8 cfu/g. University area samples had the highest average total counts. Kim et al. [78] revealed that the survey data collected by provincial centers, and hygienic and epidemiology stations in Hanoi (Vietnam) between 1986 and 1989 indicated that some street foods were of poor microbial quality. Often cold meals were contaminated with pathogenic bacteria.

Desserts/Sweetmeats

Sweetmeats are high-risk food products for microbial contamination since they are milk based. Chakravarthy et al. [62] reported that the different types of sweetmeats sold by the street vendors in Calcutta (India) such as sandesh, rasogola, jelebi and laddu showed the presence of microorganisms (standard plate counts ranging between $0.04 \times 10/g$ and $7.10 \times 10/g$), coliforms (0 and $6.2/g$), yeast and molds. Most of the sweetmeat samples sold by the street vendors in Pune (India) were free from serious contamination except for revadi, godishev, burfi, petha and kharvas. Boonyaratanakornkit et al. [87] reported that microbial contamination in the desserts sold by the street vendors in Bangkok (Thailand) was low. Some of the dessert (n = 41) samples showed the presence of *C. perfringens* (3.4%) and *S. aureus* (13.8%).

The microbial quality of the sweetmeats sold by the street food vendors in India was poor because in most of the preparations milk was used and milk has a poor microbial quality and is highly susceptible to microbial attack. However, in other Asian countries most of the sweetmeats do not use milk in their preparations.

Ice Creams

Several studies have been conducted on the microbial quality of ice creams in the various Asian countries. For example, the microbial quality of the ice creams sold by the street vendors in various cities of India such as Agra, Allahabad, Bangalore, Bombay, Calcutta, Delhi, Hyderabad, Poona, Tirupati and Udaipur has been observed by various workers since the 1940s. A summary of their results is displayed in table 9. These studies revealed that the microbial quality of the ice creams was poor. The quality of the ice cream sold by the street food vendors was also compared with ice creams sold from different sources like hotels, restaurants, factories, parlors and manufacturing units by various authors [89–94]. They reported that the quality of ice cream sold by the street food vendors was inferior because of repeated handling, unhygienic surroundings, poor quality of cups, cones, and wrappers used, sale of ice cream bars without paper wrappers, keeping the unsold ice cream overnight at higher temperature and selling it the next day, opening the ice box frequently during sales, and keeping it open over longer periods.

However, studies conducted in the early 1990s by Sarada and Begum [95] and Reddy et al. [96] revealed that microbially no significant differences were found between the samples from hotels, parlors, manufacturing units, etc. On the contrary, the samples from parlors and hotels showed higher standard plate counts when compared to local vendors (table 9). Similar observations of the ice cream samples collected from other Asian countries were also observed. Hartog et al. [69] reported that Esputer samples (a vanilla ice prod-

Table 9. Microbial quality of the ice creams sold by street food vendors in India

Place	Year	Ref. No.	Source	Type	Samples n	Standard plate count	Coliform count
Agra	1972	89	manufacturing plants and vendors	–	85	2×10^3–299×10^6/ml	0–174×10^6/ml
Allahabad	1977	97	different sources	–	168 samples each summer and winter season	0.0026–845×10^6/ml	0–22×10^5/ml
Bangalore	1991	95	local vendors	cups, cones bars lollies	120 (total number from different sources)	99.97×10^5 33.54×10^5 48.37×10^5 0.38×10^5	10,537/g 301,722/g 26/g 0
Bombay	1972	90	public hawkers, shop vendors, catering establishments	cups/bars sticks	270 (total)	$450 \times 1 \times 10^7$/ml	5–71×10^3/ml
Calcutta	1979	98	different manufacturers	cups	100	0.018×4.810^6/g	0–2,400 t/g
	1995	62	street vendors	–	–	12.30×10/g	3.83/g
Delhi	1968	91	restaurants and vendors	–	92	1×10^3–93×10^6/ml	0.840,000/ml
Hyderabad	1983	92	hotels, restaurants, parlors, local vendors	slabs cups bars cones lollies	300 31 70 25 25 150	5.106 logs 5.597 logs 5.545 logs 6.572 logs 5.793 logs	0– > 100/g
Lucknow	1956	93	vendors	–	75	0–1×10^8/ml	–
Madras	1962	94	itinerary vendors	cups and bars	30	0–270×10^6/g	0–24×10^5/g
Poona	1992	99	street vendors	ice cream kulfi ice candy ice lolly Pepsi cola	– – – – –	7.89×10^7.g (Av) 2.87×10^7/g (Av) 2.5×10^5/g (Av) 2.6×10^6/g (Av) 1.2×10^5/g (Av)	2.07×10^5/g (Av) 9.75×10^4/g (Av) 3.15×10^4/g (Av) 2.3×10^3/g (Av) 1.25×10^3/g (Av)
Tirupati	1994	96	local street vendors	cups and bars	20	250–$6,500 \times 10^2$ cfu/ml	0–4.85 cfu/ml
Udaipur	1969	100	local market	–	40	1.1–220.0 million/g	300–27×10^4/g

uct) collected from the street vendors in West Java (Indonesia) were highly contaminated with bacteria. Joshi [2] reported that the microbial quality of the ice creams sold by the street vendors in Khatmandu (Nepal) were substandard with mesophillic counts beyond the limits. The samples were also contaminated with coliform bacteria, *Salmonella*, yeast and molds. This low quality of ice creams may be due to the low quality of milk powder and the polluted water used in its preparation. According to Bryan et al. [65] the ice creams sold by the street vendors in Pakistan contained coliforms (4.2×10^5 g/ml), *S. aureus* ($< 10^2$/ml) and *B. cereus*.

Foodborne Diseases

There have been no recent epidemiological studies to suggest that street foods contribute to a significant number of food poisonings; however, there have been several documented cases of food poisoning outbreaks due to street foods [23]. Lianghui et al. [81] reported that street foods was responsible for 691 food poisoning outbreaks. 20,187 cases and 49 deaths accounting for 44.6, 43.81 and 18.2%, respectively, of the total from 1983 to 1992 in Shandong Province (China). Dawson [56] and Dawson and Canet [12] reported that in October 1988, 300 people in Hong Kong became ill following consumption of Choisum (green vegetable) which reportedly was caused by excessive pesticide residue.

In another study in 1981, a cholera epidemic in Pune city (India) was traced to contaminated sugar cane juice with added ice. The ice was found to be contaminated with *V. cholerae*. Although perhaps not completely scientific, consumers of street food in Pune city were questioned about their experience with illness following eating street foods and 12% of them reported they had had diarrhea and vomiting at one time or another after consuming street foods and 10% reported having indigestion on one or more occasion [26]. Seth [25] reported that of 75 consumers interviewed in Secunderabad (India) only 1 revealed ill-health like diarrhea/vomiting or pain in the abdomen after consumption of street foods. Chakravarthy [32] and Gandham [82] reported that in Calcutta and Pune (India) during their study in cases after consumption of street foods, discomfort, viz. stomach upset, vomiting and general dislike, was reported. Vanchianathan [101] reported that the Calcutta press had published data on food poisoning episodes caused by the consumption of hawker foods from 1984 to 1988; the number ranged from 0 to 5 and the total percentage was 7.4. Isolated reports of foodborne diseases due to consumption of street foods were being reported in daily newspapers in India. These include (1) death of 5 people and hospitalization of about 100 after consuming sweetmeats from wayside stalls in the Nizamabad district of Andhra Pradesh (India) [102]; (2) two persons developed nausea and vomiting after eating ice cream from a roadside vendor in Hyderabad city [103]; (3) falling ill of about 100 children after consuming ice cream sold from a pushcart by a vendor in Nandyal and surrounding villages, Andhra Pradesh (India) [104]. Waghray and Bhat [44] reported one death due to food poisoning and development of symptoms like vomiting and diarrhea in 41 others after consumption of *idli* from a street vendor in Srungavarapukota, Vizianagarm due to accidental contamination of the *idli* by the pesticide endosulfan. Such newspaper reports are very common. When the recorded hospital data were screened for the outbreak none were due to street foods. Most of the incidences where foodborne disease outbreaks occurred were after the consumption of stale food (19%), biryani (14%), stale biryani (11%), and milk-based sweets (9.5%) [105].

Perdigon [3] reported that during the period of the study, a food poisoning case occurred in the state of Ipoh (Malaysia) where 12 children died after eating *mee*, a type of rice noodle prepared locally by the Chinese. A newspaper report indicated three areas of contamination – chemical, microbial and natural toxins from plants. The government directed health officials to intensify checks on food factories and street food hawkers. It was found later that the samples of Loh shee fun rice noodles consumed by the victims had boric acid as a component (as noted earlier, boric acid is used illegally to bleach and give a shine to the noodles). Another view for the cause of death of the above 12 children was not because of boric acid but it was suspected that the toxicity was induced by the consumption of contaminated food (food containing afla-toxin B_1). The liver tissues of the above patients were analyzed and they revealed the presence of AFB_1 adducts which strongly suggests aflatoxin poisoning leading to acute liver failure [106].

Of 135 street foods in Iloilo (Philippines) only one item caused diarrhea among the study participants [16]. Lim [107] reported that in metro Manila (Philippines) during July to September 1989, 158 people suffered from a cholera outbreak which was due to the consumption of pansit from the street food vendors which was contaminated by *V. cholera*. In Singapore, there were 25 notifications of cases of food poisonings during 1987. This represents 0.3% of the total number of food vendors [6, 12, 23, 56]. Unhygienic and unsafe foods causing intestinal diseases are one of the most common factors causing consumer deaths in Vietnam. From 1987 to 1990 there were 1,707 cases of food poisoning in Vietnam, of this number 70 persons died [7].

HACCP (Hazard Analysis Critical Control Points)

HACCP is intended to make food protection programs evolve from a mainly retrospective quality control toward a preventive quality assurance approach and to provide an increased confidence in food safety. It involves four basic components: (1) identification and assessment of hazard; (2) deter-mination of critical control points essential to control any identified hazard; (3) establishment of appropriate systems to monitor critical control points (CCP), and (4) verification that the system is working effectively providing information on its performance. These components are basic 'functions' or 'missions' the system must perform whenever it is intended to use HACCP at the production, processing, manufacturing, packaging, storing, transforma-tion, and distribution stages until the point of consumption.

Several studies have been conducted in the Asian countries pertaining to the Hazard Analysis Critical Control Points of different kinds of street foods

[108]. Dayue et al. [109] worked on the application of an HACCP system in cooked meat products such as stewed chicken, pig head and beef cooked in soy sauce in China. The critical control points for the different meat products were identified as follows: (a) Stewed chicken: The main source of hazard from stewed chicken was microbial contamination after cooking. The cooked products were contaminated by unsanitary containers, utensils, or hands of food handlers in the course of transport storage and selling. (b) Stewed pig head: The critical control points were similar to stewed chicken. In addition, some special CCPs such as the temperature and the time of reheating were identified. The products were inevitably contaminated at the bone picking step after cooking in unsanitary containers or utensils or hands. (c) Beef cooked in soy sauce: The CCPs were similar to stewed chicken. Additional CCPs identified were avoiding the use of synthetic color and industrial dye stuff that is on the surface of the cooked meat.

In another study in China, the critical points at which contamination can occur in street foods were identified in different types of foods, e.g. cooked meat products, Chinese style salads and various types of stalls (mobile and night markets) using the HACCP approach [49].

Chakravarthy [32] and Chakravarthy et al. [62] conducted HACCP studies for different street foods sold by the street vendors in Calcutta (India). The critical control points for different foods like sandesh (water and the cheese-cloth used for washing and staining), egg rolls and ghuni (got contaminated while being kept at the vending table in the street food stall), and water (duration of storage and frequency of handling; the bacterial quality of water deteriorates progressively over the sequence, i.e. from municipal water to the drinking water offered by the vendor to the customer) [62].

Hema et al. [57] also conducted HACCP studies of some street foods sold in Coimbatore. They reported that the CCPs of plantain bajji were handling procedures and display before sale. HACCP studies for sugar cane juice sold by the vendors in Hyderabad were also conducted. The results revealed that the critical control points were the extraction of juice with the help of equipment, the ice added to the juice, glasses used, and the water used for washing [84].

Hartog et al. [69] applied the HACCP concept to improve the quality of street foods commonly sold in Indonesia. He reported that CCPs for different food preparations were: (a) Nasi rames: a mixed rice dish – improper handling of cooked rice stored in open pans and addition of insufficiently reheated leftovers. (b) Esputer: a vanilla ice product which often had poor microbial quality. Preparation procedures of the dough and coconut milk components are the main crucial points. (c) Gado-gado: a dish containing steamed or blanched vegetables highly contaminated with bacteria particularly through bad handling and improper storage of vegetables. (d) Escendol: a beverage consisting of sago dough lumps. 'Cendol' mixed with coconut milk and sugar syrup and added shredded ice generally contained a high number of bacteria. CCPs were in both the preparation of cendol and coconut milk. Stoots et al. [77] also reported that application of the HACCP concept proved to be very useful to evaluate the composition, preparation and handling of street foods suspected to be hazardous. They developed some simple recipe modifications and adjustments of preparation methods, reducing the microbial contamination for some selected street foods in Bogor (Indonesia).

Desmachelier [110] conducted the HACCP analysis for the street foods sold by hawkers in Malaysia. He identified prolonged ambient temperatures and storage of food as a major critical control point. Several studies have been conducted by Bryan and his team on the HACCP analysis of different types of street foods from various locations in Pakistan. The hazard analysis of ground meat, chicken (fresh), rice pattis and ice cream sold by the vendors in a mountain resort town in Pakistan revealed that cutting boards, knives, hands of the vendors and the wiping cloth were the CCPs [65].

The CCPs of a chat (a regionally popular food in Pakistan) were handling after cooking and holding on display [66]. Hazard analysis of commonly sold street foods such as rice, pulses, chickpea, ground meat and okra at railway and bus stations in Pakistan revealed high temperature holding or periodic reheating as the CCPs [31].

Kim et al. [78] conducted the HACCP studies of some popular street foods sold in Hanoi (Vietnam). The CCPs of some of the foods were (a) mixed rice dish (raw vegetables, poor handling practices, use of dirty dishes, utensils and contaminated water); (b) ice cream (preparation of the mixed dough, sugar cane syrup and other components); (c) lunar sweet cake (poor packaging and handling such as exposing the ingredients to dirty tables, utensils and storage containers).

Later a document was developed by WHO for the governments entitled 'Street vended food: A HACCP-based food safety strategy for governments' which deals in detail with how to conduct the HACCP analysis practically in the field to determine critical control points. The HACCP concept was applied to street foods in 23% of the countries which participated in WHO street-vended food survey [111].

Legislation

Studies conducted with regard to legislation in the Asian countries have revealed that there is no uniformity among countries as to licensing system, legislation, requirements of vendors to possess licenses, health certification, etc. The street food activity was not recognized or regulated in many countries but was merely tolerated or ignored until the vendors became a nuisance. Scattered information on these aspects is available from various Asian countries. Bhat [34] reported that in India regulation of street food by local government agency has not been attempted except in a few selected instances. Municipal Corporation of Madras has attempted a regulation on urban street foods. In Maharashtra, street food vendors were provided licenses on the same terms and conditions as regular eating establishments. In Andhra Pradesh, no systematic attempt has been made to register, issue licenses or regulate street foods. Chakravarthy [32, 112] reported that though India has fairly comprehensive regulations on food, the Indian penal code, municipal acts (e.g. Calcutta municipal acts in Calcutta), prevention of food adulteration acts, the public health departments of the government, the municipal corporations and the police administer regulations for ensuring quality and safety of food. However, street foods always being taken as a passing phase and being despised by the local administration never got enough attention from the enforcing agencies and have not been controlled and also do not come under any of the above regulations.

In Korea to date, the street food vendors (Ponjangmacha) have no legal status and there is no systematic control over them in terms of law and sanitation [7]. In Yangon city of Burma (Myanmar), street foods were regulated under Rangoon Municipal Act of 1922 (reformed recently as the Yangon City development act). This act prescribes in accordance with its bylaws, the control and supervision of the selling of the food along the sides of the streets and roads throughout the city. It also includes the inspection and sanitary regulation of milk sellers, bakeries, public eating houses, refreshment stalls, water and ice-producing places [7].

Perdigon [3] reported that street food hawkers in Penang are regulated by the local government act of 1976 of which embodies the hawkers, 'bylaws of 1979', the market bylaws 1980, and food handlers bylaws of 1983. In Sri Lanka under section 31 of the Food Act 1980, there was a provision to issue regulations to enable all premises dealing with manufacturing, distribution and sale of food including street foods to be registered with the relevant food authority. The basis of registration was the code of hygienic practice for the preparation, storage and sale of foods approved in 1988 under the provision of the act. However, the implementation of this code was delayed as the necessary regulations have still not been issued [7].

Possession of the license by the street food vendors varied from country to country. In Kaula Lumpur there are 28,478 vendors of which only 12,000 are licensed. In contrast, in Singapore there are 23,331 vendors who are licensed and every vendor involved in food cooking is required to be vaccinated against typhoid. Those that are 45 years of age and older are also required to be tested every 3 years for tuberculosis [113]. In Malaysia, there are 40,434 registered hawkers. In urban areas hawkers are registered or licensed by local authorities while those in rural areas are licensed by the ministry of health [7]. In Mynmar (Burma) also street vendors possess license [7].

While in China the studies revealed that 67.8% of the food vendors were legal and 32.3% were illegal and at the time of completion of the studies the percentage of legal vendors reached 100% [49]. In Secunderabad, only 2 vendors of 133 had obtained a license for hawking food items from the municipal corporation [25].

In Pune, licenses were issued to individuals intending to sell street foods by the Pune Municipal Corporation authorities under certain fixed rules and regulations. Depending on the type of sale, different types of licenses were issued. About 1,100 different types of license were either newly issued or renewed since 1984 onwards. As per the conditions laid down, street food sellers holding licenses were subjected to inspections at intervals [26].

Harassment of street food vendors by government officials is common in all the Asian countries and the incidents are no longer news. About 63% of hawkers in Secunderabad (India) complained of harassment from local traffic police, or anti-encroachment staff of the municipal council, while one hawker also complained of seizure of a food sample by the food inspection staff and some others indicated interference from food inspectors.

Various studies conducted in the different countries of the Asian continent revealed that the vendors are not aware of the details of the PFA act (Prevention of food adulteration act), basic sanitation, and hygienic requirements [6]. For example, in Secunderabad (India) 60% of the vendors were not aware of the provisions of the PFA act, while 30% of them were aware of the need for maintaining food hygiene [25]. Similar observations were made by Bharathi [30] in Hyderabad city. The vendors were not aware of standard weights and measures in terms of unit number of pieces, permitted food coloring, artificial colors, and food laws, which regulate the quality of foods being sold. The process of licensing in the different Asian countries is a time-consuming procedure and most of the vendors are unaware. In Malaysia, the process of licensing requires the hawkers to comply with specific health requirements such as medical examination and sanitary provisions. The rationale for medical examination was more psychological in nature hoping that contact with the health procedure would create awareness of the relationship between health and food and also provide an opportunity to impart some health education to the licensee [7].

The insecurity engendered by the threat of government harassment was cited as the major problem faced by the vendors in the Asian countries. In order to overcome this, in Iloilo (Philippines) vendor's associations have been formed in an effort to reduce confrontations with the police. In return for self-policing to ensure that the vendors did not sell in front of any store which objected, did not occupy more than half the pavement, and kept the surroundings clean, the police reduced their harassment. A seminar conducted by the Equity Policy Center was attended by association heads. They, along with major persons in the seminar, discussed other mechanisms to improve both the situation of the vendors and the appearance of the town [28].

In Manikgunj (Bangladesh), a local social service group tried to help organize the vendors. They met with the town and district officials during the EPOC seminar to discuss some ways to legitimize the vendors by the bus stop and along the main roads leading into the court area [28].

Government is also undertaking various measures for the street foods in the different Asian countries [7, 114]. In Vietnam, the government is preparing a strategy for food protection and safety. Though there is no code of practice for street foods, some related issues were being taken into account in laws and regulations [7]. In Thailand, some guidelines are being implemented for the street food vendors [7]. In Indonesia, at the national level, the street food sector has been a matter of concern among several authorities or the various authorities. Under the Ministry of Health, initiatives have been taken to establish an interdepartmental forum with its main objective being to promote coordination and communication on street food activities undertaken by each party. Legal provisions are there to ensure proper standards of food but these are not adhered to in Bangladesh. The Pure Food Ordinance had given power to the municipal authorities to seize food considered to be adulterated or impure. The Dhaka Municipal Corporation has 20 positions for inspectors to enforce the provisions of the said ordinance (Pure Food Ordinanace, 1959) but at present only 9 sanitary inspectors are working to inspect and examine the quality of food [7]. In the regulation of street foods in Nepal, the agencies involved were the District Administration Office, the municipality, the police and the solid waste management office. There are 6 consumer associations and one hawker association in Nepal [7].

There is a network of food inspectors in each city in Vietnam, with 4–22 inspectors. The government of Vietnam organized some national training workshops and seminars for food inspectors, and food safety and control for its food inspection and health staff, but the street food hawkers, helpers and food handlers have not been provided with training in food hygiene.

The concern over the implications for health of the consumers of street foods has been reflected in the continuing strong interest in the elaboration of a draft code of hygienic practice for the street foods under the guidance of the Codex Alimentarius Commission [115]. The draft was viewed as a guide for hygienic practices for the countries of the region to be adapted to a variety of local conditions. It also recognized that special sociocultural practices do exist in the regions and that appropriate additions and adaptations should be introduced, and along with this a clear interest in regional, subregional and even national peculiarities, and recognition of the importance of 'core elements' and core codes [58].

In Sri Lanka, the government will establish in the near future a new code similar to the proposed draft code of practice for hawker food by Malaysian authorities and present it to the 8th session of Codex Coordinating Committee for Asia [7].

Bhat and Waghray [116] prepared a draft code containing a series of requirements and practices to be followed in the preparation and sale of street foods and drinks for direct consumption and submitted it to the Municipal Corporation of Hyderabad (India). Dawson et al. [117] reported that in Thailand, the Department of Health developed a ten-step code of practice for street food operators.

Kits have also been prepared for testing street foods. In China, the Sino American Joint Venture Huayan Power and Electronics Technology Development Co. Ltd. of Shenyang developed a kit 'Materials used in quick proof to street foods'. The 'quick proof to street foods' is an effective means by which varieties of foods and dinner sets could be supervised in order to keep them sanitary. The materials can both make a rough estimation of food hygiene, distinguish between real and false, estimate the quantum, and check the effect on disinfecting foods and dinner sets, especially giving a qualitative and quantitative analysis of the coli group. The materials would become effective checking tools.

Urban street food is bound to increase in the near future in all the Asian countries. Besides enacting and enforcing legislation, it is necessary to improve the hygienic practices.

(1) Earmarking certain places for selling of street foods in congested commercial areas and along streets.

(2) Providing basic facilities like electricity, water, trash cans, waste disposal, sewage disposal. Courses should be offered to vendors on sanitation and nutrition and those vendors who get through this course should be given access to prize spots near cinemas, school grounds, etc.

(3) Organizing vendors into associations to make the administration easy. Credit facilities should be made available for the vendors. Evolve a uniform licensing system in a country.

(4) Maintain close scrutiny of the food safety aspects including nutritional, microbiological and adulterants. Preparing food safety educational materials and launching proper education of the food handlers/vendors with the appropriate extension network.

References

1   Krishna KV, Ghosal SC, Banerjee R: Bacterial standards for ice-cream. Indian Med Gaz 1944;79: 423–425.
2   Joshi U: Street foods in Nepal; in Natarajan CP, Ranganna S (eds): Trends in Food Science and Technology. Mysore, Association of Food Science and Technologists (India), Central Food Technological Research Institute, 1995, pp 771–776.
3   Perdigon G: Assessment of the economic impact of street foods in Penang. Rome, Malaysia Food and Agriculture Organization of the United Nations, 1990, pp 1–88.
4   Bok TK: Street Food Improvement and Control in Singapore. Working Paper Expert Consultation on Street Foods, 5–9 December 1988 Yogyakarta, Indonesia. Rome, Food and Agriculture Organization of the United Nations, 1988, pp 1–15.
5   Chen LH, Chen SK, Liu TY: Street foods in Taiwan. Abstracts – Street Foods Epidemiology Management and Practical Approaches, Beijing, Oct 19–21, 1993, pp 28–29.
6   FAO: Street Foods. FAO and Foods and Nutrition Paper No 46. Rome, Food and Agriculture Organization of United Nations, 1990, pp 1–30.
7   Anonymous: Street foods in Asia. Second FAO Regional Workshop, Kuala Lumpur, Malaysia, 24 January 1992, pp 1–26.
8   Abdussalam M, Kafferstein FK: Safety of street foods. World Health Forum 1993;14:191–194.
9   Battcock M: Street foods and development in Bangladesh. Food Lab News 1992;8:14–22.
10   Wedgewood H, Jones A, Battcock M: Feeding whose needs. Appropriate Technol 1994;20:1–3.
11   Chapman B: Street foods in Indonesia: Vendors in the urban food supply. Chevy Chase MD, Equity Policy Center, 1984.
12   Dawson RJ, Canet C: International activities in street foods. Food Control 1991;2:135–139.
13   Aziz H: Hawkers' food in Malaysia: A reevaluation. Proc First Asian Conf Food Safety. The Challenges of the 90s, Kuala Lumpur, Sept 2–7, 1990, pp 135–138.
14   Webb RE, Hyatt SA: Haitian street foods and their nutritional contribution to dietary intake. Ecol Food Nutr 1988;21:199–209.
15   Cohen M: The influence of street food trade on women and child health; in Jelliffe DB, Jelliffe EFP (eds): Advances in International Maternal and Child Health. 1986, vol 6, pp 148–165.
16   Winarno FG, Allain A: Street foods in developing countries: Lessons from Asia. Food Nutr Agric 1991;1:11–18.
17   Winarno FG: Street foods in developing countries: Lessons from Asia. Abstracts – Final Programme Street Foods Epidemiology, Management and Practical Approaches, Beijing, Oct 19–21, 1993, pp 2–3.
18   Chakravarty I, Canet C: Street foods in Calcutta. Food Nutr Agric 1996;17/18:30–37.
19   Allain A: Street foods: The role and needs of consumers. Working Paper for the Expert Consultation on Street Foods. Yogyakarta, Indonesia, FAO, 1988.
20   Hubies IAVS, Pajaaran JR: The role of local government in street food development in Indonesia. Abstracts – Street Foods Epidemiology, Management and Practical Approaches, Beijing, Oct 19–21, 1993, pp 40–42.
21   Tinker I: The case for legalizing street foods. Ceres 1987;20:26–31.
22   Barth GA: Street foods: Informal sector food preparation and marketing in the Philippines. Iloilo City, Equity Policy Center, 1983.
23   FAO: Street foods: A Summary of FAO Studies and Activities Relating to Street Foods. A Report. Rome, Food and Agriculture Organization of the United Nations, 1989, pp 1–28.
24   Gayathri K, Rani PJ: A study on the extent of adulteration with food colours in the street foods of Anantapur; MSc thesis, Sri Sathya Sai Institute of Higher Learning, Anantapur, India, March 1993.
25   Seth R: A profile on street foods in Secunderabad; MSc Diss, Andhra Pradesh University of Health Sciences, 1990.
26   FAO: Study on street foods in Pune India. Pune, Food and Agriculture Organization of the United Nations and State Public Health Laboratory Pune, Government of Maharashtra, India, 1986, pp 1–133.

27 Hutabarat LSR: Street Foods in Bangkok: The Nutritional Contribution and the Contaminants Content of Street Foods. Rome, Food and Agriculture Organization of the United Nations, 1994, pp 1–179.

28 Tinker I: Street foods. Current Sociol 1987;35:1–110.

29 Anon: Grameen Bank Annual Report, Shyamoli Bangladesh, 1986.

30 Bharathi S: Consumption of street foods by urban population and their safety; MSc thesis, Andhra Pradesh Agricultural University, 1995.

31 Bryan FL, Teufel P, Riaz S, Roohi S, Quadar F, Malik Z: Hazards and critical control points of vending operations at a railway station and bus station in Pakistan. J Food Protect 1992;55:534–541.

32 Chakravarthy I: Urban street foods in Calcutta. Abstracts of Scientific Sessions of 27th Annual Meeting of the Nutrition Society of India, National Institute of Nutrition, Hyderabad, India, November 24–25, 1994, p 6.

33 Jadhav JNR: In vitro digestibility of proteins and contents of trace elements of street foods consumed by slum dwellers; MSc thesis, Marathwada Agricultural University, 1996.

34 Bhat RV: Urban street foods: A challenge to regular catering establishments. ACP Newslett 1991; 1:4–6.

35 Atkinson SJ: Street foods; in Moleolo B (ed): Food for the Cities. Urban Nutrition Policy in Developing Countries. London, PHP Departmental Publication, London School of Hygiene & Tropical Medicine, 1992, No 5, pp 37–38.

36 Kaur N: Household food preservation and processing in Malaysia. 1st Asian Household Nutrition Appropriate Technology Conference, Colombo, July 13–17, 1981.

37 Club du Sahel: La Stretegia Alimentarie du Mali. Ministère de l'Agriculture, Republique du Mali, 1982.

38 Jellinek L: The Life of a Jakarta Street Trader. Center for Southeast Asian Studies, Working Paper No 9, Monash V Australia 1978.

39 Tinker I, Cohen M: Street foods as a source of income for women. Ekistics 1985;52.310:83–89.

40 Wang Z, Zhang H, Chen B, Shang J, Shen Z: Approaches for assuring the safety of street foods. Final Programme/Abstracts Street Foods Epidemiology, Management and Practical Approaches, Beijing, Oct 19–21, 1993, p 26.

41 Zhenhu G, Zhonghua H, Pengjiang G, Jining S, Xilan L, Ling L: The hygienic control of street food in Shaanxi Province. Abstracts Final Programme Street Foods Epidemiology, Management and Practical Approaches, Beijing, Oct 19–21, 1993, pp 30–31.

42 Li-guo QI, Zhang Y: The hygienic conditions of street food in Yinchuan city and some relevant suggestions for improvement. Abstracts Street Foods Epidemiology, Management and Practical Approaches, Beijing, Oct 19–21, 1993, pp 22–23.

43 Waghray K, Bhat RV: Studies on ready-to-eat traditional foods marketed in streets of Hyderabad in Regional Workshop on Indian Traditional Foods at CFTRI-Regional Centre, Sept 19–20, 1996. Mysore, Ministry of Food Processing Industries, Government of India and Central Food Technological Research Institute, 1996, pp 30–31.

44 Waghray K, Bhat RV: Street foods of Hyderabad: A profile. Nutrition 1995;29:11–23.

45 Kulkarni AP: Food quality control and processing. Eating on the run. Food Lab News 1992;8:10–13.

46 Anon: Vital statistic Peninsular Malaysia 1987. Kuala Lumpur, Department of Statistics, Kuala Lumpur City Hall, 1989.

47 Pothisiri P, Liamrangsi S: Street food and urban development in Thailand. Abstracts Final Programme Street Foods Epidemiology, Management and Practical Approaches, Beijing, Oct 19–21, 1993, pp 22–23.

48 Waghray K, Bhat R: Street foods sold on special occasions in Hyderabad, South India. 1996;unpubl.

49 FAO: Pilot study on improving the safety of urban street foods in China. NU 12/43 PRC-FINAL REPORT. Food and Agriculture Organization of the United Nations. Beijing, Institute of Food Safety Control and Inspection, Ministry of Public Health, 1993.

50 Prakash A: Rehri – The mobile shops in India. Ekistics 1972;34.204:328–333.

51 Li-guo QI, Zhang Y: The hygienic conditions of street foods in Yinchuan city and some relevant suggestions for improvement. Abstracts – Street Foods Epidemiology, Management and Practical Approaches, Beijing, Oct 19–21, 1993, pp 22–23.

52   Andring K, Kier Y: Street Food Hawkers in Southeast Asia. Utrecht, 1989.
53   Kiran TU: Quality characteristics of snack foods sold near school in twin cities of Hyderabad and Secunderabad; MSc thesis, Andhra Pradesh Agricultural University, 1987.
54   Devdas RP, Easwaran P, Aruna M: Impact of educating the roadside catering vendors on health, nutrition and sanitation. Abstracts – Final Programme Street Foods Epidemiology, Management and Practical Approaches, Beijing, Oct 19–21, 1993, p 10.
55   De Guzman MPE: Improvement of street food quality and safety through training. Abstracts – Street Foods Epidemiology, Management and Practical Approaches, Beijing, Oct 19–21, 1993, p 49.
56   Dawson RJ: International activities on street foods; in Merican Z, Ahamad N, Queean Y, Moy MG, Othman NDM, Shahabudin MA, Mohamed AR (eds). Proc 1st Asian Conf Food Safety: The Challenges of the 90s, Kuala Lumpur, Sept 2–7, 1990. Malaysia, Malaysian Institute of Food Technology, 1990, pp 129–134.
57   Hema MS, Chandrasekhar V, Kowsalya S: A study on selected street foods of Coimbatore. Abstracts Scientific Sessions Nutrition Society of India, XXVI Annual Meeting, Nov 24–25, 1994, p 15.
58   Dawson RJ: FAO and street foods. Proc 3rd World Congr Foodborne Infections and Intoxications, 16–19 June, 1992. Organized by Institute of Veterinary Medicine Robert Von Ostertag Institute FAO/WHO Collaborative Centre for Research and Training in Food Hygiene and Zoonosis, Berlin, 1992, pp 802–805.
59   Khan TS: Nutritional evaluation of the selected junk foods consumed by slum children of Parbhani City; MSc thesis, Marathawada Agricultural University, 1995.
60   WHO: Essential safety requirements for street vended food. 1992. Doc WHO/HPP/FOS 92.3. Geneva, WHO (provisional).
61   Abdulssalam M, Kaferstein FK: Essential approaches to the safety of street foods. Proc 3rd World Congr Foodborne Infections and Intoxications, 16–19 June, 1992. Organized by Institute of Veterinary Medicine Robert Von Ostertag Institute FAO/WHO Collaborative Centre for Research and Training in Food Hygiene and Zoonosis, Berlin, 1992, p 801.
62   Chakravarthy I, Canet C, Roy BR: The present status and control of microbial foodborne diseases in street foods of Calcutta; in Natrajan CP, Ranganna S (eds): Trends in Food Science and Technology. Mysore, Central Food Technological Research Institute, 1995, pp 777–789.
63   Bhat RV, Waghray K, Jonnalagadda P: Interim report on urban street food in Hyderabad and Secunderabad. Hyderabad, National Institute of Nutrition, 1994, pp 1–32.
64   Grover MR: Street foods in India: Their control and inspection. Working Paper for the Expert Consultation on Street Foods, Yogyakarta, 1988.
65   Bryan FL, Teufel P, Riaz S, Roohi S, Quadar F, Malik Z: Hazards and critical control points to street vending operations in a mountain resort town in Pakistan. J Food Protect 1992;55:701–707.
66   Bryan FL, Teufel P, Riaz S, Roohi S, Quadar F, Malik Z: Hazards and critical control points of street vended chat, a regionally popular food in Pakistan. J Food Protect 1992;55:708–713.
67   Barrot P: Green packaging: Local biodegradable and its even edible. Ceres 1995;27:9–10.
68   Dumo NS: Street foods. Nutrition 1985;19:3–11.
69   Hartog BJ, Stoots JAM, Heryanto B, Fardiaz B, Fardiaz S: Application of the HACCP concept to improve the safety of street foods. Food Lab News 1992;8:23–39.
70   Smith A: Pests and vectors in an urban environment. Working Paper Joint FAO/WHO Expert Consultation on Food Protection for Urban Consumers, 1–5 December 1986. Rome, Food and Agriculture Organization of the United Nations, 1986.
71   Boutrif E: Global perspectives of street foods; in Natarajan CP, Ranganna S (eds): Trends in Food Science and Technology, Mysore. Association of Food Science and Technologists (India), Central Food Technologists Research Institute, 1995, pp 753–759.
72   Wirakartakusumah A: Development of a street food push cart that meets HACCP requirements. Abstracts – Final Programme Street Foods Epidemiology Management and Practical Approaches, Beijing, Oct 19–21, 1993, pp 58–59.
73   Anonymous: Meeting the transport needs of poor people with cycles and tractors. Appropriate Technol 1994;20:IT News 3.
74   Seth R, Bhat RV: Study on Urban Street Foods in Secunderabad: A Report, 1991, pp 1–43.

75 IDRC International Development Research Centre: Hawkers and Vendors in Asian Cities, 1975, pp 1–23.

76 Liang YM, Yuan XS: Investigation of bacterial contamination of street vended foods. Dairy Food Envir Sanit 1991;11:725–727.

77 Stoots JAM, Heryanto B, Fardiaz D, Hartog BJ: Application of the HACCP concept to improve the safety of street foods. Proc 3rd World Congr Foodborne Infections and Intoxications, June 16–19, 1992. Organized by Institute of Veterinary Medicine Robert Von Ostertag Institute FAO/WHO Collaborative Centre for Research and Training in Food Hygiene and Zoonosis, Berlin, 1992, p 926.

78 Kim PH, Duc BM, Yen PT: HACCP and the study of food processing and street foods in Vietnam: Survey of Hygiene Quality of Street Food in Hanoi. Abstracts – Final Programme Street Foods Epidemiology, Management and Practical Approaches, Beijing, Oct 19–21, 1993, pp 24–27.

79 Vatanasuchart N: Chemical contaminant in street foods. Food 1994;24:35–41.

80 Santos RV, Udarbe MA, Reyes GD, Garcia RG, Bungay AC, Lozada AF: Nutritional quality and safety of selected street foods: Barbecued and deep fried animal by-products. Abstracts – Final Programme Street Foods Epidemiology, Management and Practical Approaches, Beijing, Oct 19–21, 1993, p 24.

81 Lianghui X, Xingling SM, Yuju C, Zhang L, Haiyan W: Analysis of street food safety in Shandong Province. Abstracts – Final Programme Street Foods Epidemiology, Management and Practical Approaches, Beijing, Oct 19–21, 1993, p 15.

82 Gandham SV: Study of street foods in Pune with special reference to chemical analysis (artificial sweeteners, colouring agents, and bacteriological analysis for palatability (MPN counts); Thesis, BJ Medical College, Pune, 1994.

83 Chandrasekhar U, Kowsalya S: Nutritive value and microbial quality of selected street foods of Coimbatore and nutritional knowledge of vendors. Abstracts – Final Programme Street Foods Epidemiology, Management and Practical Approaches, Beijing, China, Oct 19–21, 1993, p 6.

84 Nagalakshmi AVD: Quality analysis of selected fruit juices sold by street vendors in Hyderabad; MSc thesis, Andhra Pradesh Agricultural University, 1995.

85 Kaul M, Aggarwaal G: Microbial load of common 'chat' products. Ind J Nutr Diet 1988;25:197.

86 Pillai RAV, Khan MMH, Reddy VP: Incidence of aerobic spore formers in lassi. J Food Sci Technol 1993;30:141–142.

87 Boonyaratanakornkit M, Anage P, Huan S, Thamawat P, Stansaovapak S, Panpeng B: Microbiological quality of street foods in Bangkok. Food 1993;23:35–43.

88 Guha AK, Roy R, Das HN, Roy BR: Bacteriological quality of cucumber slice and its public health significance. J Food Sci Technol 1983;20:245–247.

89 Bathla JM, Rao YS: Studies on the microbial quality of ice cream in Agra city. Ind J Dairy Sci 1972;24:254–256.

90 Thatti BL, Gayakwad KS, Laxminarayana H: Survey of the quality of ice cream in Bombay market. Ind J Dairy Sci 1972;25:9–13.

91 Rao RS, Natarajan AM, Dudani AT: Bacteriological quality of ice cream sold in Delhi market. Ind J Dairy Sci 1962;15:39–44.

92 Rajalakshmi: The microbiological quality of ice creams sold in Hyderabad city. J Food Sci Technol 1983;20:19–20.

93 Govil KK, Bhatnagar DP, Pant KC: Nutritive and hygienic qualities of ice cream. J Ind Med Assoc 1956;27:245–249.

94 Ray B, Vedanarayakam AR, Varma K: Bacteriological quality of ice cream in Madras city. Ind Vet J 1962;39:361–367.

95 Sarada M, Begum JM: The microbiological quality of ice creams sold in Bangalore city. J Food Sci Technol 1991;28:317–318.

96 Reddy BBB, Reddy YK, Ranganadham M, Reddy VP: Bacteriological quality of ice cream marketed in Tirupati, a pilgrimage town of India. J Food Sci Technol 1994;31:151–152.

97 Singh A, Singh RB, Edward JC: Study on the microbiological quality of ice cream in Allahabad city. Ind J Dairy Sci 1977;30:167–169.

98 Guha AK, Das HN, Roy R, Devan ML: Microorganisms in ice creams and their public health significance. J Food Sci Technol 1979;16:161–164.

99 Sagade RB: Study of street foods in Pune; in Bhat RV, Rao RN (eds): Proc National Workshop on Food Safety in Public Catering, National Institute of Nutrition, Hyderabad, Nov 1–3 1989. 1992, pp 59–70.

100 Pagaria ML, Saraswat DS: Studies on the bacteriological quality of ice cream in India. Aust J Dairy Technol 1969;24:200–203.

101 Vanchianathan S: Laboratory support service in food safety: Microbial contaminants – Current status and regulations; in Bhat RV, Rao RN (eds): Proc National Workshop on Food Safety in Public Catering, National Institute of Nutrition, Hyderabad, Nov 1–3, 1989. 1992, p 115.

102 Anonymous: Five die after taking adulterated foodstuff. The Hindu 1993, April 27, Tuesday.

103 Anonymous: Two persons ill. The Deccan Chronicle, 1994, vol 57, No 73, 15th March.

104 Anonymous: 100 kids taken ill after eating ice cream. Indian Express, 1995, 12th February.

105 Rao RN, Sudhaker P, Bhat RV: A study of recorded cases of foodborne diseases at Hyderabad during 1984 and 1985. J Trop Med Hyg 1989;92:320–324.

106 Harrison JC, Garner RC: Immunological and HPLC detection of aflatoxin adducts in human tissues after an acute poisoning incident in SE Asia. Carcinogenesis 1991;12:741–743.

107 Lim QC: Cholera in Metro Manila (street food consumption leads to cholera). Abstracts – Street Foods Epidemiology, Management and Practical Approaches, Beijing, Oct 19–21, 1993, pp 13–14.

108 Bryan FL: Hazard analysis of street foods and considerations for food safety. Dairy Food Envir Sanit 1995;15:64–69.

109 Dayue B, Maoqi W, Li T, Xifang L: Studies on application of HACCP system in street foods (cooked meat products) control. Abstracts – Street Foods Epidemiology, Management and Practical Approaches, Beijing, Oct 19–21, 1993, pp 38–39.

110 Desmarchelier PM: Ensuring microbial safety of street vended food. Abstracts Final Programme Street Foods Epidemiology, Management and Practical Approaches, Beijing, Oct 19–21, 1993, pp 56–57.

111 World Health Organization: Street vended food: A HACCP based food safety strategy for governments. WHO/FNU/FOS/95.5, 1995, pp 1–22.

112 Chakravarty I: Management of street foods in Calcutta. Final Programme Street Foods Epidemiology, Management and Practical Approaches, Beijing, Oct 19–21, 1993, p 5.

113 Goerge J: Towards more organized street vending in Kuala Lumpur. Proc 1st Asian Conf Food Safety. The challenges of the 90s, Kuala Lumpur, Sept 2–7, 1990, pp 139–142.

114 Costarrica ML: Practical approaches to improve street foods at the municipal level. Abstracts Final Programme Street Foods Epidemiology, Management and Practical Approaches, Beijing, Oct 19–21, 1993, pp 54–55.

115 FAO/WHO: Draft code of hygiene practice for the preparation and sale of street foods. Joint FAO/WHO Food Standards Programme Alinorm 91/15 Appendix III. Rome, Food and Agriculture Organization of the United Nations, 1990.

116 Bhat RV, Waghray K: Minimum requirement for the preparation and sale of street foods: A draft code. Hyderabad, National Institute of Nutrition, 1994, pp 1–16.

117 Dawson R, Liamrangsi S, Boccas F: Bangkok's street food project. Food Nutr Agri 1996;17/18: 38–45.

Dr. Ramesh V. Bhat, National Institute of Nutrition, Indian Council of Medical Research, Jamai-Osmania P.O., Hyderabad 500 007 AP (India)
Tel. +91 40 7018909, Fax +91 40 7019074, E-Mail nin@ap.nic.in

Simopoulos AP, Bhat RV (eds): Street Foods.
World Rev Nutr Diet. Basel, Karger, 2000, vol 86, pp 100–122

....

Street Foods in Africa

Ramesh V. Bhat, Kavita Waghray

National Institute of Nutrition, Indian Council of Medical Research,
Hyderabad, India

Historical Aspects

Among the agricultural tribes of the African continent, the women used to sell the surplus of agricultural produce up until the colonial period. Later, the British colonial authorities encouraged male migration to mines and cities, at the same time prohibiting them from bringing their wives and families [1]. This separation of households created an urban demand for prepared foods and traditional beer which women prepared and supplied throughout the region specially in Eastern and Southern Africa [2, 3]. After World War II, the policies changed and women were allowed into the town, but the wages for men were too low so the women entered the trading business. They were allowed to trade only with Africans because it was illegal to trade with Europeans.

In post-independence Africa, some of the women started moving up from farm produce and prepared foods of higher status commodities like fish, as well as provisions, hardware and eventually textiles. For example, in Zambia and along the coast of West Africa and Senegal women purchase and prepare dry/smoked fish and sell them, and some of them are involved in the network of moving these products deep into the deserts [4, 5]. In Zambia, women specialised in the preparation and marketing of cooked foods along with other household goods. The women used the income to feed and clothe their families and educate their children [6].

Unlike in Asia, in Africa economics often makes street foods cheaper, convenient and more time saving than foods prepared at home, especially in view of the high cost of cooking fuel, the drudgery, and the long preparation time. For example, maize needs dehulling and grinding, cassava needs shredding and drying, soybean needs fermenting to save hours of boiling: monie,

a millet-based gruel, needs to be simmered for a long time. Similarly, bean-based foul and tamia, and millet-based cous cous also need hours of preparation [7, 8]. The fuel costs are also very high in most African countries, e.g. Nigeria. Traditional foods eaten at home often take hours to process and require lots of cooking time and fuel. Busy housewives or working women avoid this effort by feeding their families street foods. For example, in Dakar (Senegal) 32% of the families eat millet cous cous for their evening meal, only 12% of the urban women actually prepare it at home and the rest purchase from street vendors [9]. However, in Egypt the basic diet of cheese and bread is served cold, so that meals require a minimum preparation time.

Most African countries are dependent on agricultural produce for their livelihood. Studies in Ghana indicated that a good maize harvest results in a low maize price (300 cedis to 25 cedis/tin) which is accompanied by increased cooking at home and decreased demand for prepared street food [8, 10]. In contrast, studies in Nigeria indicated that a recession period was accompanied by an increase in street food trade as food items became scarcer on the markets, and fuel costs rose [11]. Thus, eko (corn pudding) and stew were substituted for home-cooked rice dodo or yam, all of which are increasingly costing more [11]. Household surveys indicated an increase in the consumption of street foods. This may be because of difficulty in obtaining foodstuffs and cooking materials like fuel, etc. Street food vendors prepare in bulk enabling the food to be cheaper [7, 12].

Peoples choice of food depended both on culture and levels of modernization. For example, Nigeria had a strong market economy for centuries so it was not surprising that almost everyone seemed to eat at least some of their meals on the street [13]. The strength of an eating out tradition is also a key variable affecting the level of street food demands. It is strong in Nigeria where both the Muslims in the north and the Yoruba in the west have a well-entrenched tradition of eating street food snacks and meals [8]. In Minia, Egypt, the number of street food enterprises is increasing faster than the increase in city size. A possible explanation for the exception of Minia lies in the types of food eaten as a regular diet.

Socioeconomic Aspects

The street food industry is a vast business which falls into the category of the invisible economy of the country. In Rabat (Morocco) street food sales reached 90×10^6 Dirhams (1 USD = 9 Dirhams) [14]. The relationship of price to quantity of food is significant; by eating street foods, consumers were able to obtain their daily requirements for about 18 Dirhams [15].

Expenditure

The expenditure on street foods by the people varies from place to place in different African countries based on income, traditions, culture, etc. Consumer surveys indicate that street foods are eaten by people in all income groups and everyone spends about the same percentage on such foods, i.e. the amount spent on street foods rises along with the income. In Ile-Ife (Nigeria), one third of the funds spent on foods goes for street foods. Students (46%) and informal sector traders (38%) are the largest consumer groups, both of which represent various income groups followed by white collar workers (11%) and others (5%). In Zigunchor (Senegal), there is a slight variation: students (35%), followed by others (31%), white collar workers (24%), and informal sector (10%) being the main consumer group of street foods [13, 16]. The majority of the consumers (78.3%) in Kampala (Uganda) spent 10,000–15,000 units of the local currency (=USD 10–15) per month on street foods followed by 9.8% who spent between 5,000 and 10,000; 9.5% spent over 5,000 and only a few (1.7%) spent less than 5,000 per month for purchasing street foods [17].

Food Budget

In Ile-Ife (Nigeria) as much as 50% of the food budget was spent on street foods while in Senegal it was estimated to be 15–20%. This lower level of demand in Senegal was attributed to the small size of the city which ensures a close proximity between work and home. Similar observations were also made in Hausaland [8].

However, a variation exists between different residential areas as to the percentage of household food budgets that go for street food in Central Ife. In the mixed residential/commercial area, over half of the budget is spent on prepared foods near the campus. In the older residential areas, families spend only a third of their budget on street foods [7]. In African countries, breakfast was the most important meal bought from the street vendors. For example, household surveys in Ile-Ife (Nigeria) showed that 83% of the people buy their breakfast from vendors on an average between 4 and 7 days a week. An even higher percentage (96%) eat breakfast on their way to school.

Number of Persons in the Street Food Business

The street food trade is hard work. More than three quarters of vendors in Africa showed a one-man enterprise, although they might have had unpaid family help at home. The largest one-man enterprises were found in Africa. For example, 95% in Zigunchor and 84% in Ile-Ife, Nigeria. Unpaid family labor at the point of sale, usually the spouse but also children and parents, is present. In general, about 10% of the enterprises have paid employees to help with the selling. The average persons per enterprise were 1.7 in Minia (Egypt) but most of the additional labor was by unpaid family members [7].

Income of Street Food Employees
The employees of the street food vendors in Kampala (Uganda) were rather poorly paid, the majority (87.7%) were given below 9,000 (USD 9.00) per month even though all of them fed on street foods [17].

Franchise
In African countries, the street food vendors acquire money to start their business from different sources. In Ile-Ife, almost all the vendors (91%) started their business either with money from their own savings or from relatives. While the remaining 10% of the cases received interest-free loans from their friends. Money lenders were not a significant source for starting a business. Another method of starting without their own funds was to get an advance from a producer or distributing company (e.g. Coca Cola). But such facilities were not available to the vendors in African countries. Daily credit for foods prepared and sold on the day was also common. Forty-four percent of vendors in Minia (Egypt) used this type of credit. No interest was charged on these foodstuffs, but many vendors thought that their costs would be reduced if they could buy in greater quantities [7].

Role of Women
Studies conducted on street foods in some African countries revealed an increase in the employment of women ranging from 40 to 95% in the street food operations not only in the preparation and serving of food, but also in marketing [18]. Less than 50% of street food vendors are women in some regions of Senegal, while they form 53% in Zigunchor (Senegal) and 72.5% in Kampala (Uganda) [8, 17]. In some places like Ile-Ife and Ibadan (Nigeria), the percentage increases up to 95% [18]. In Senegal, yoghurt which was made from fresh milk was sold by women only; they did not use imported dried milk powder as in the preparation used by male vendors [19]. Mostly traditional foods and those foods whose consumption is increasingly being advocated by policy makers as well as nutritionists were sold by women [8]. Since women spend more time at home, they spend less time selling in the streets. For example, women vendors spent 4–5 h compared to 7–8 h of vending a day by men. The women prepared a set amount of food (which took a longer time to prepare and also spent time on household activities), sold it and returned home. It is not clear whether they could make and sell more considering the preparation time. There is also some indication that women had less access to new foodstuffs [19]. Women who were fully employed in the street food

enterprises were relieved of their home tasks by other family members [10]. The provision of day care is often mentioned in those countries where young women were vendors [20].

A strategy of food self-sufficiency was observed among women in African countries. For example, all women in Hausa (North Nigeria) saw that their families ate three meals a day, but virtually no women cooked three meals a day. Most of them purchased 2 out of 3 meals a day from other women or 'door-step vendors' i.e. street food vendors who set up a table and chair on the sidewalk outside their home or hawk foodstuffs at a nearby corner or directly in front of their door [21].

In no country were women found selling on commission; only men who sold ice cream in Zigunchor (Senegal). Although there is an overlap of food sold by females and males in 3 or 4 African countries there is some sex specificity in the mode of selling. For example, no men were observed selling out of the baskets which could be carried on one's head, conversely no women were observed pushing a mobile cart [19].

Women had lower incomes compared to men and also the seasonal variations influenced their income. In Zigunchor though women vendors earned (370FCFA) more than housemaids (250FCFA) their income was low when compared with women in other parts of Africa. For example, in West Africa market women earned a very good income, often more than their civil-servant husbands [8, 19]. In some African countries women were economically independent. For example, in Zigunchor (Senegal) 59% of the women were sole or major providers for their families which have an average size of 9.5 people [19]. Even in Minia (Egypt) women vendors (55%) provided the main source of income but men (70%) also did so. Income earned by women goes more directly to support the household, children's education and as a means to secure a better income than the income earned by men.

Profile of Street Vendors

Number of Vendors
The number of street food vendors in the different African countries varied from country to country (table 1). This variation in the population was related to the total population, food and cultural habits, etc. The ratio of vendors to total population varied from 1:52 in Nigeria to 1:255 in Egypt (table 2).

Age
There was a wide variation in age of the street food vendors in the African countries. Most of the vendors were between the age group of less than 20–45

Table 1. Population/census of street food vendors in Africa

Country	City/town	Number of street vendors	Ref. No.
Egypt	Mania	784	7
Ethiopia	Awassa	50	22
Nigeria	Ile-Ife	2,603	13
Senegal	Zigunchor	1,534	7
Uganda	Kampala	490	17

Table 2. Ratio of vendors to total population in Africa [7]

Country	City/town	Total population	Total number of street vendors	Ratio
Egypt	Mania	2,000,000	784	1:2550
Nigeria	Ile-Ife	1,350,000	2,603	1:520
Senegal	Zigunchor	86,295	1,534	1:56

years. In Zigunchor (Senegal), Ile-Ife (Nigeria) and Minia (Egypt), the vendor's age ranged between 30 and 45 years while in Kampala (Uganda), the majority (88.9% of 490 vendors) were between 20 and 45 years of age, 4.7% were less than 20 years and 6.4 were greater than 45 years.

Educational Level

Educational level among vendors varied across the continent of Africa. Illiteracy is presumed to characterize vendors and this is indeed the case in Zigunchor 80%, Ile-Ife (60%) and 93% in Minia (Egypt). In Minia, 47% of the men had some schooling and 17% had graduated from secondary school [7]. In Kampala (Uganda) most of the vendors had some formal education: 63.8% had primary education and 26.4% had post-primary and only 9.8% had no education at all. Less than 2% of the vendors had some formal training in food handling [17].

Migration Pattern

Several interesting facts stand out from the data on the migration of street food vendors in African countries. Street food vendors are not recent migrants of the cities in the African countries. Even among those who were not born in the town, most had lived there for over 10 years. Increased rural poverty does not require migration. Many of those vendors born in rural areas near the city continue to live there, and commute daily to work in the city [7]. In contrast, in Minia (Egypt) only 3% of the vendors currently live in rural areas, so there has been migration from these areas to that city. However, 28% of these vendors in Minia (Egypt) commute from other urban areas in the Minia governorate while 29% listed their birth place as urban areas in Minia or Clippert (Nigeria). This means that of the current vendors living in the city, 80% were born in the city, another 5% came from other urban areas, and 15% came from rural areas [7]. Street food is not the sole source of income of the families. The vendors have their own farms, e.g. in Ile-Ife 7% of the vendors maintained farms.

Religion

There is a wide variation in the vendor's religion in the different African countries. In Kampala (Uganda), Christians were in the majority (81.5%) compared to 15% Moslems and 3.5% others. This distribution is rather similar to the distribution of the Ugandan population by religion nationally, rather than the concentration of Christians in Kampala city [17]. In Kampala (Uganda) almost all the vendors (99.4%) were Ugandan nationals while 0.6% were non-Ugandan. Of these, 41.6% came from the western, 37% from the central, 11.4% from the eastern, and only 9.2% from the northern part of the country [17].

Marital Status

Marital status of the street vendors in African countries varied from place to place. In Kampala (Uganda), of 490 vendors 34.5% of them were living alone, 56.5% were married, and 9.0% were widowed [17].

Number of Customers Catered

The number of customers catered by a vendor during the day and in the peak business hours varied from vendor to vendor and from city to city. In Minia (Egypt), a street vendor caters a minimum of 60 customers per day [13].

Number of Business Years

In the most urbanized country, Egypt, vendors are urban born, while data suggest a high failure rate in the early years of an enterprise. Street vending was a permanent occupation for many. In Zigunchor 20% of the vendors sold the same product in the same place for over 20 years [7]. In Kampala (Uganda) 59.7% of the vendors had spent less than 5 years selling while 41.6% had spent longer. This also indicates that as time progresses, vendors eventually become secure in their respective places of business [17].

Peak Business Hours/Days

The peak business hours and days of the street food business varies from vendor to vendor and place to place in the different African countries. Nasinyama [17] reported that the peak business hours were at lunch time (63.7%) followed by evening (19.7%) and morning (6.1%), as well as non-specific times (10.5%). Similarly, the peak business day was Monday (42.2%) with most of the customers followed by Tuesday (16.7%), Friday (12.0%), Wednesday (10.7%), Thursday (8.3%) and the rest of days were less than 6%.

Income

Studies conducted in some African countries like Nigeria and Morocco have shown that street food vendors usually earn more than the country's minimum wage [16]. In Nigeria, 74% of the vendors made equivalent to or more than the minimum wage [18]. The income of the majority of the street food vendors in Kampala (Uganda) (8.7%) grossly ranged between 5,000 and 20,000 (about USD 5–20) a day with only 8.9% getting less than 5,000 – while a small percentage (3.9%) gets over 20,000 per day. When comparing the street food vendor's income with the minimum government wage in the civil service per month, i.e. 5,000 (about 240 per day), none of the food vendors interviewed earned below the minimum wage [17]. In Ile-Ife, the data collected during the recession period reveals that about half the vendors were making meagre profits with only a quarter making a good income [7].

Profile of Consumers

Age

Unlike in Asian countries, there is a variation in the age group of consumers from infants to 40 years in the African countries. In some African countries, the use of street food begins in infancy. For example, in Zigunchor, yoghurt is frequently given to babies as a weaning food and is never prepared at home [8]. In Nigeria, 70% of the consumers were between the ages of 10 and 40 years. Students under 20 years of age constitute 21% of the consumers [18]. In Morocco, 60% of the street food consumers were aged less than 30 years [15] while in Kampala (Uganda) the age of consumers who consumed street foods ranged from 16 to 35 years [17].

Educational Level

In African countries, the majority of the consumers have a minimum of primary school education. For example, in Nigeria and Senegal, schoolchildren are the major consumers of street foods. In Kampala (Uganda), the majority of consumers (92%) had at least a primary school education. Of 952 consumers 36.7% had a primary school education, 42.5% had secondary and 12.8% had post-secondary school education. Only 8% of the consumers were illiterate.

Sex, Religion, Marital Status

Though many studies have been conducted on street foods in different African countries, detailed information regarding the sex, religion and marital status of the consumers is not available except for the study conducted in Kampala (Uganda). The majority in Kampala were males (76.4%) only 23.6% were females. Christians were the dominant group of consumers (86.6%) with Moslems accounting for 11.5% while others were 0.8%. Among the consumers 39.3% were married, 57.5% were living alone, and 3.2% were widowed [17]. In Morocco, 60% of the consumers were single [15].

Type of Consumer

The majority were schoolchildren followed by other categories. In Nigeria, consumers were schoolchildren and adults. The study also revealed that 53% of the consumers are in the lower socioeconomic strata [18]. In Kampala, the majority of the consumers were petty traders, civil servants and students followed by farmers, professionals and others [17]. In Zigunchor (Senegal) and Ile-Ife (Nigeria), the majority of the customers were children (35%) or students 46%. In Zigunchor, 24% of the customers belonged to the white-collar group, while in Ile-Ife 11% belonged to the white-collar group and 5% were others [13].

Number of Meals Purchased

General statistics on consumers have shown that in Nigeria most consumers visit food vendors during breakfast and lunch periods. The majority of the consumers (71%) eat only one meal per day from street food vendors. Increasingly, street food vendors have become a major source of food for schoolchildren [18]. A study conducted on Nigerian schoolchildren revealed that 8% of the children who bought street foods purchased one street food meal, 76% purchased two meals, and 16% purchased three meals daily [19]. In another study, it was also observed that 96% of the Nigerian school students bought breakfast from the vendors before the start of the school day [23].

Intake of Nutrients

In some countries, this source for the first half of the day is important to the student's daily diet [24, 25] and provides proteins and vitamins which are not readily obtainable in any other form [26]. Although the nutritional contributions of such meals and snacks to the diet of school student's is substantial, its significance is often overlooked in food consumption survey efforts [26]. Street foods were the major source of nutrients for many of the adolescents ($n = 142$) in Abeokuta (Nigeria). Between 40 and 70% intake of all the major sources of food groups were obtained from street foods which were the major source of dairy products (70%), legumes (60%), fish (50%), meat (50%) and eggs (50%); 21% of energy for males and 29% energy for females was supplied by street foods. Street foods also supplied greater than 50% total proteins, 64% calcium and 60% vitamin A for both males and females. For other minerals (iron) and vitamins (thiamine and ascorbic acid) street foods supplied greater than 50% of total intake [27].

Choice of Street Foods

In Morocco, 30% of the consumers were buying street food on a daily basis [14]. In no study was it shown that consumers chose a particular food for its nutritional value. In Nigeria, the taste of the food was the primary reason. Generally, the next most popular reasons for selecting street foods were their low cost, followed by their convenience/availability. In Kampala (Uganda) consumers gave various reasons for the selection of street foods. Of 942 consumers: 24.9%, taste; 24.6%, price; 22.6%, nutrition; 13.5%, satisfaction; 1.2%, hotness.

Selection of Vendor

Selection of a particular vendor by consumer varied from person to person and place to place. In Kampala (Uganda) the reasons given by the consumers for selecting a particular vendor are convenient location (15.6%), good food (10.7%), cleanliness (25.8%), regular customers (25.0%), kindness (18.8%), and large amount of food 4.0% [17].

Profile of Street Foods Sold

Variety

A variety of street foods breaking the monotony of diets are sold in the different African countries depending upon tradition and culture [17]. In Ethiopia [6], Egypt [11], Kampala [23] and Ghana [33] several varieties of street foods were sold. Unlike in Benin and Senegal, they were as many as

Table 3. Type of street sold in different African countries

Country	Name of the street food dish	Ref. No.
Benin	fermented cooked corn flour, corn flour cooked in water, corn bread, boiled rice, macaroni with sauce, sieved and precooked manioc, manioc fritters, boiled beans, bean fritters, sauces (tomato, oil, meat, vegetables), pasta, smoked fish and shrimp fried fish, hard boiled eggs, fried turkey, gari	28, 29
Egypt	rice boiled, fried rice, oriental rice, rice and vegetable, Kushari, rice and shirea, tamia, foul, Egyptian salads (single item, two items and three items), tahina, meat, meat organs, viscera, macaroni, spaghetti, desserts, cheese, pickles, olives, barley water, dates, bean dishes	13, 30–32
Ethiopia	roasted offals, fish soup, cooked and sauced macaroni and spaghetti, Shiro sauce, pancake-like yera or bread	22
Ghana	(gari) roasted cassava dough, fish (fried and smoked fish), sugar, rice, beans, pito, palm wine, iced kenkey, hausa beer, Akpeteshie, tiger nut milk, pastries, confectionary, fula, fried plantains and yam, fanta, pap, kenkey, ga kenkey, abolo, apitsi, fufu, agidi, estew, bread, fried meat (chicken, turkey, pork), groundnuts (fired and roasted), popcorn, ice lollies, Nmadaa	8, 33
Nigeria	eko, stew, rice dodo	7
Senegal	meals, kababs, postoral-peuhl, monie, yoghurt, fresh brochettes, fish fry, cous-cous, nuts, soups	7
Uganda	mandazi, roasted chicken, fried fish, chapatti, roast meat, pancakes, potato roast, roast Nsenene, simsim balls, oluwombo, kitobero, malewa, eshabwe, katogo, pillawo, malakwang, obusuman, engeni, cassava chips, roast maize, groundnuts, popcorn, soybeans, ice cream	17

126 and 129. Included were: soups, salads, snacks, sweetmeats to full-course meals, as well as alcoholic and nonalcoholic beverages (table 3). One common feature of street foods in Africa is that the prepared foods are usually based on the staple and traditional foods consumed in each country. Two products made from dried beans, foul and tamia, are very popular in Egypt. Soups and meals are also sold in different parts of the world but their ingredients vary. Noodles with bits of fish or vegetables predominate in Nigeria and the base is farina [13].

Seasonality

Seasonality is a major feature in the African countries. At the time of harvest, many vendors come from the cities to their family farms to assist in planting and harvesting the crop and later in the off season they go back to the cities for street food vending. In Zigunchor (Senegal), the total number of vendors fell to less than half from 1,534 in the dry season to 748 in the rainy season. Similar observations were also observed with female vendors [7].

Source of Procurement of Raw Materials

The source of procurement of raw materials varied from vendor to vendor and country to country in Africa. In Kampala (Uganda), most of the food vendors (94.1%) procured their raw materials for food preparation from markets in the morning on a daily basis, while 5.9% of the vendors got food from farms.

Type of Fuel Used

Very little information is available from African countries regarding the type of fuel used by street food vendors. In Kampala (Uganda), of 490 street food vendors 81.2% used charcoal, 17.3% used firewood, while 1.4% used electricity. In this study, 77.6% of the vendors spent between 500 and 1,000 of their local currency for the fuel per day.

Storage of Raw Materials and Containers Used

The storage of raw food materials by street food vendors varies from vendor to vendor in most of the African countries. This depends on whether the food is prepared at home or on site and the amount of space available. For example, in Kampala (Uganda), street food vendors stored raw food materials both at the street food business location and at home. They were stored on the floor, in a sack, nylon bags, metal tins, baskets, plastic containers, cupboards, fridges, under water, etc. [17].

Place of Preparation and Processing Methods

Data on these aspects are very meagre. In Kampala (Uganda) 79% of the street vendors prepared the food on the street and only 21% prepared it at home. While 88.4% of the vendors prepared different snack items once, 4.7% prepared in batches, and only 7.0% prepared on demand. The types of dishes prepared by vendors depicts the tribe and tradition of consumers. A vendor is not limited to one tradition in order to attract as many consumers as possible [17]. Ashenafi [22] reported that in Awassa (Ethiopia) some of the food items like spaghetti or macaroni were cooked and sauced at home and bought to the market (vending site) to sell, by the vendors, while roasted offal, fish soup and shiro sauce were prepared at the vending place.

Storage, Serving, Display Containers

There is a variation in the serving storage and display containers/materials used by the street food vendors in Africa. In Kampala (Uganda), street food vendors stored cooked food in different containers made of plastic, earthenware, millet containers, i.e. traditionally woven baskets with covers, glass, metal containers and also wrapped in leaves (banana) and nylon materials [17]. In Uganda, prepared food was mainly kept warm on a fire (79.8%) covering (20.2%) it with various materials like banana leaves or plastic bags [17].

In Awassa (Ethiopia) street food items like cooked and sauced spaghetti or macaroni were displayed on vending tables in large uncovered trays [22]. No information on the various types of serving containers and serving methods used by the street food vendors in Africa is available.

Packaging Materials

A variety of packaging materials have been used by the street food vendors in Africa. In Ghana, street food vendors used old jars and bottles, cane baskets, newspapers, polythene pouches, leaves (plantain, T-populnea, marantoclea), sheaths of maize and multi-wall portland cement sacks, old stationery waste, etc., for packaging [33]. In Kampala (Uganda), street vendors used banana leaves, plastic bags and paper as packaging materials [17]. Due to the ill/adverse effects caused by the modern non-biodegradable packaging materials like plastic bottles, polythene bags, etc., the era of 'green technology' in the packaging has entered into the African markets. Traditional biodegradable packaging materials made of leaves or jute are entering the markets. Different types of leaves are used in Africa as packaging materials. They are the biloria leaf (*Crytosperma senegalense*) used to wrap 'Chicouanges', banana, taro, sugarcane or *Thaumatococcus* leaves used to wrap, cook and transport food products, and papaya leaves used to wrap meat [34].

Leftover Food

Very meagre information is available regarding the leftover food in Africa. In Kampala (Uganda) most of the vendors did not have cooling facilities and whatever food remained unsold, they carried home and consumed it.

Water Source

Among the most critical problems is the lack of an adequate supply of potable water for cooking, cleaning, cleaning of mixing and eating utensils, personal hygiene, use in beverages, and as drinking water [14]. In most cases potable water was not available from the city taps and in some places, e.g. Ibadan (Nigeria), the flow was usually intermittent being available only for a few hours daily or within 1 week. Vendors in such locations used water from different sources which are usually heavily contaminated. In order to save water, these vendors economise by not using hot water for cleaning the utensils; equipment and dishes were washed in the same water all day without being changed. Water was not used for personal hygiene. This resulted in poor environmental sanitation. Thus, the food as well as water becomes contaminated making it unsafe for consumption [18]. In Ile-Ife, only 8% of the street food enterprises had access to running water. While other sources were questionable, 69% of the vendors used shallow well water, 3% used stream water, 12% bought from water vendors, and a few used rain water [7]. In Kampala (Uganda), tap water (from the Municipal supply) was the major source (63.5%) used in food preparations followed by spring water (29.7%). An observation made here was that due to the erratic nature of the water supply by the municipality, vendors normally purchased water from the water vendors whose source may be unknown. However, there are a number of springs around Kampala, some of which have been protected by local authorities. In addition, water is normally used sparingly by food vendors resulting in the same dishwashing water being used over and over again for cleaning utensils and even plates for the consumers [17].

Waste Disposal

Very meagre information on the system of waste disposal by street vendors in Africa is available. Nasinyama [17] reported that in Kampala (Uganda) the local authorities were ensuring garbage removal from markets where street foods were sold. In Awassa (Ethiopia) the intestines and stomach parts of the animals were cleaned and their contents were disposed of within only 2 meters of the cooking area [22].

Location

In Senegal and Nigeria, the street food vendors clustered where the customers were present. They were found along the roads, near cinema halls, schools, hospitals, bus stops, train stations, in stalls or near the markets. They also collect in narrow down-town streets. The majority of street food establishments were also found outside the commercial areas like in Ile-Ife (Nigeria). The number of street food vendors increases with city size [7, 13].

Type of Vending Vehicles

In most of the African countries, the truly mobile vendor is in the minority. Most carts are pushed to the same location each day and removed at night. Some vendors have two regular positions, e.g. school and cinema. Even women selling from baskets carried on their heads tend to squat in the same place everyday; in front of the court, next to the bus station or outside the market place. There are some really mobile vendors using bicycle carts to pedal bread or sate or ices. Also used are shoulder balance poles with a tiny stool to be carried on one side to balance the sweets or tea held on the other. Such vendors follow a regular route everyday. These mobile vendors accounted for a quarter of all sellers in Ile-Ife (Nigeria) and 10% in Zigunchor (Senegal) [7].

In Kampala (Uganda), there were two types of shelters: open type of street food vending locally known as 'Toninyira Mukange', and closed type. The common means of transport for foods prepared at home to the market place were wooden carts, pickups, motorbikes, bicycles and in some cases actual carrying on heads in locally insulated vessels [17]. In Senegal, yoghurt was sold as a street food from large calabashes by women sitting on the ground outside the market place. Similarly, soups were also sold by women. Women also sold nuts from baskets which they carry on their heads. In Senegal, heavy pushcarts were usually the province of men who position them at the same intersection everyday to sell meat chunks of larger size popularly called kabab [7]. In Awassa (Ethiopia), street food vendors prepared and served food in small temporary shelters of approximately 9 m^2. These had a capacity to accommodate about 10 people to be served at a time [22].

Materials Used in Construction of Vending Vehicles

Materials used in the construction of vending vehicles depend upon the place, climate and economic status of the vendors. In Kampala (Uganda), the commonest materials used in the construction of eating kiosks were papyrus, mats and poles [17].

Quality of Street Foods

Physical Quality

Information on quality of street foods include nutritional value, microbiological qualities and food additives. However, no analyses were done for physical quality parameters like filth, dust particles, soil, insects, and animal contamination. The data dealing with the descriptions of location and sites of vending reveal that a considerable amount of contamination from afore-mentioned sources could be possible. The habit of exposure of street foods by the vendors in Kampala in open receptacles especially in the open type of food vending predisposes to a high risk of contamination by dust flies and other vermin [17]. Dishes containing rice in different cities of Egypt were exposed to dust, flies, insects, etc. [30]. Cooked and sauced spaghetti and macaroni samples prepared by the street food vendors in Awassa (Ethiopia) were exposed to dust, flies, and insects as they were not covered while being displayed. A large number of flies were also observed around the vending shelters [22].

Chemical Quality

Though many studies have been conducted on street foods in the various African countries, no detailed information on chemical quality and nutrient content of the street foods is available.

Nutritional Quality

The nutritional investigations carried out in Nigeria revealed that freshly cooked traditional street foods are a source of nutrient [35]. It was also believed that many low income families would be worse off if there were no street foods [36]. Street foods have been regarded as nutritious and often superior in quality to their industrially manufactured counterparts. For example, comparison of unit nutrient costs of different cereal breakfasts consumed in Kenya revealed a 10:1 price difference between the cheapest traditional staple (maize flour 100% extraction) and an imported breakfast cereal [37].

Microbial Quality

The street foods sold in different African countries in general were of poor microbial quality. Street food samples such as cheese and roast chicken sold by the street vendors in Ibadan (Nigeria) showed the presence of *Salmonella* [18]. Most of the street samples sold by the street vendors in Kampala (Uganda) were safe microbiologically. However, some foods sold along pavements like mandazi (half cakes) showed the presence of *E. coli* (52 cfu) and *Streptococcus* (45 cfu); roasted chicken, pancakes contained *Streptococcus* (18 cfu); chapathi also contained *E. coli* (35 cfu) and *Streptococcus* (25–40 cfu); Nsenene showed the presence of *E. coli* (40–45cfu); roast meat had *E. coli* (15–35 cfu); cassava chips had *E. coli* (12 cfu), *Streptococcus, Shigella* and *Salmonella*. It was also observed that cold foods showed the presence of pathogens while hot foods were free of pathogens [17].

In Awassa (Ethiopia) spaghetti and macaroni kept at ambient temperature (20–30 °C) had high aerobic mesophillic counts (>10 cfu/g) and enterobacteriaceae counts (>10 cfu/g) and also yielded *Shigella* and *Staphylococcus* species. Most of the other food items were held at higher temperatures (>40 °C) and the aerobic mesophillic counts in most cases was relatively lower ($<10^5$ cfu/g). Several bacterial genera were also isolated. *Micrococcus* and *Bacillus* species dominated the aerobic microflora. In the unhygienic conditions of the food service environment, the possibility of cross-contamination from utensils and keeping food items at ambient temperatures for several hours were considered to be the critical points [22].

Ice Creams

Ice cream samples collected from the street vendors in Ibadan (Nigeria) showed the presence of *Salmonella* [18]. In Kampala (Uganda), vanilla and strawberry ice cream were positive for *Klebsiella* and *E. coli*, respectively. Strawberry ice cream could have been contaminated during packaging while in vanilla ice cream *Klebsiella* organisms might have survived pasteurization. Contamination might have occurred because of the large number of cows that were suffering from a particular type of mastitis. On the other hand, the fluid milk pack did not show any microbial activity [17].

Snacks

Among the food samples (n = 126) from fermented cooked corn flour in water, corn bread, boiled rice, macaroni with sauce, sieved and precooked manioc, manioc fritters, boiled beans and bean fritters, sauces (tomato, oil, meat, vegetables), pasta, smoked fish and shrimp, fried fish, hard boiled eggs and fried turkey collected from street vendors in Benin (West Africa), around 60% of the samples were of poor quality. Out of the total samples 24.3% were of good quality, 15% were acceptable, 25.3% were poor quality, 29.3% were not acceptable and 6.1% were dangerous. Fish and sauces were of poorest quality. *Salmonella* was absent in 100% of the food samples but high levels of *Proteus mirabilis, Pseudomonas aeruginosa, P. fluorescens* and *Providencia stuartii* were present [28].

Food samples (n = 114) such as meat organs and edible viscera, fish, rice, dishes containing rice and raw vegetables, salads, macaroni, spaghetti, cheese, bean dishes, dates, tahina (sesame paste), pickles, olives and barley sugar water collected over a period of 3 years from the street food vendors in Egypt were of poor microbial quality. *Shigella* was isolated from one green sample and from tamea (deep fat fried whipped beans and parsley). Coliforms were detected in white cheese, soft cheese (with pepper and tomatoes), boiled milk, rice with milk and barley water. Most of the samples that contained coliforms had counts exceeding 10^3/g, 41% of the samples were positive for *Staphylococus aureus*, 58% of them had counts at least 10^3/g. Four of 15 samples of cooked meat, meat organs and edible viscera contained *Clostridium perfringens*, 37% of the samples of rice and dishes containing rice and macaroni/spaghetti, and beans dishes showed the presence of *Bacillus cereus* and half of them had counts up to 10^3/g or greater, 68% of the samples had aerobic colony counts that exceeded 10^6 cfu/g, 97% of the samples were within the temperature range of 15–45 °C at the time of sample collection [32].

Meals

Rice dish samples sold by the street food vendors and star hotels in Alexandria, Aswan, Cairo, El-Fayoum, Giz, Hargada, Ismalia, Luxor, Port

Said, Suez and many small cities and villages throughout Egypt were of poor microbiological quality. Out of the 15 samples collected from street vendors, 13% showed the presence of *S. aureus* greater than $10^3/g$ and 43% showed the presence of *B. cereus* of which 33% of the samples had $> 10^3/g$ [30]. Tests conducted for the street food samples in Minia (Egypt) for bacterial contamination indicated that only one quarter of enterprises vending the foods were judged safe [7]. The food samples such as vegetables, fish, and meat products brought from traditional street vendors in Mercato market, Addis Ababa (Ethiopia) were of poor quality. Microbial analysis of the samples revealed the presence of enterotoxigenic strains of *E. coli, Enterobacter, Serratia, Klebsiella, Aeromonas, Pseudomonas* and *Citrobacter* [38].

The biological profile and holding temperatures of food samples/items like roasted offals, fish soup, cooked and sauced macaroni and spaghetti and shiro sauce revealed that spaghetti and macaroni were kept at ambient temperature (20–30 °C) and had high aerobic-mesophillic counts ($> 10^6$ cfu/g) and enterobacteria counts ($> 10^5$ cfu/g). These samples yielded *Shigella* and *Staphylococcus* sp. Most of the other food items were held at higher temperatures (> 40 °C) and the aerobic mesophillic count in most cases was relatively lower ($< 10^5$ cfu/g). Several bacterial genera were isolated among which *Micrococcus* and *Bacillus* sp. dominated the aerobic microflora. Staphylococci were isolated only from spaghetti and macaroni and *Pseudomonas* and *Alcaligens* sp. were isolated from cooked offal and fish soup. Unhygienic conditions of the foods service environment, possibility of cross-contamination from utensils and keeping food items at ambient temperatures for several hours were considered to be the critical points [22].

Water

The water samples collected from the traditional street food vendors in Mercato market, Addis Ababa (Ethiopia) revealed the presence of enterotoxigenic strains of *E. coli, Enterobacter, Serratia, Klebsiella, Pseudomonas* and *Citrobacter* [38].

Desserts

Starch-containing desserts sold by the street food vendors in Egypt showed positive tests for the presence of *Bacillus cereus* [32]. Raw vegetables and salad sold by the street vendors in Egypt were of poor microbial quality. Out of 30 salad samples collected 93% of the samples had aerobic colony counts $> 10^6/$ g and *Shigella* was present in one sample of parsley leaves [31].

Foodborne Diseases

In Senegal, more than 200 cases of foodborne disease were reported and, according to newspaper reports, street foods made from dairy products were incriminated as the possible source for the disease outbreaks [39]. There was a cholera epidemic in Guinea (West Africa) in 1986 resulting in more than 150,000 cases and 20,000 deaths. Detailed studies demonstrated that in this epidemic many cases of severe cholera were associated with eating specific cooked foods with *Vibrio cholerae* within the household. No increased risk was found to be associated with eating in restaurants or at vendor stalls, with the type of water used for drinking or bathing or with consumption of ice or iced drinks [40].

Legislations

Legalizing street foods in third-world countries must surely be a priority for anyone concerned with equitable development. In July 1984, the new military government in Nigeria reactivated a law forbidding structures to be built close to major roads [13]. In order to regulate vendors selling on campus, the University of Ife (Nigeria) had developed a 'bukatareia system'. The University supplies buka (stall) with water and electricity for a nominal rent to vendors who have completed a course on nutrition and sanitation run by Olumfemi Kujore of the nursing department [7].

Governments try to control street vending by requiring/issuing licenses, but too often the procedures are so time consuming that few vendors apply. For example, in Egypt a food vendor must submit a series of certificates indicating good health, no criminal record, approval of the location from the local police station, and health approval of utensils. In addition, the applicant must submit two photographs and a birth certificate and pay a fee. Even so, most of the favorite street foods are not allowed to be sold by vendors. Despite these regulations two-thirds of the vendors in Minia (Egypt) held health certificates. In contrast, another law requires stationary vendors to pay for the space they occupy but such permission is seldom granted [7].

Recommendations

Several suggestions have been provided by various authors for the improvement of street foods [7, 12, 13, 17, 22, 30, 32, 41, 42]. These are summarised below.

The essentiality of street food as seen through the enormous number of people being served and the nutritional value of the trade, coupled with its potential to offer employment opportunities and its significant contribution to economic developments, clearly indicate that it would not be possible to prevent the sale of street foods. It is generally recognized that all governments in Africa should officially recognize the socioeconomic and nutritional significance of street foods and regard the trade as indispensable in the circumstances. National governments need to take advantage to organize and assist the trade to upgrade its performance through training and development initiatives. Organizing vendors into associations would make the administering of this microenterprise easier. Such organizations should also provide a convenient channel for the provision of other services. In order to effectively improve the quality, safety and nutritional value of street foods, an integral approach involving all relevant government departments, vendors and consumers needs to be followed.

National or regional workshops for decision makers of municipalities need to be organized to create awareness and understanding of the importance of street food industry. Legislation and regulation which are predominantly educative and less punitive need to be prepared and enforced to provide for an appropriate street food handling code of practice. A system of regular spot-checks by trained personnel needs to be established to correct unsanitary conditions and assist the vendors to accept and use improved hygienic practices.

Local authorities need to create mini markets/food parks, allocate suitable sites, and provide public conveniences, water stand pipes, refuse skips and means of waste water drainage. The initial costs of providing these items may appear as an extra cost but in the long run the continuous revenue collection from vendors will ultimately sustain the authority. The most important tool in improving quality of street foods is personal hygiene and sanitation education. Arrangements need to be made for short courses of food handlers and talks about food hygiene, hygiene of service, and personal hygiene, i.e. care for the hair and nails, clothes and hand washing. There is an urgent need to educate vendors about the hazards and practical measures essential for food safety such as temperature control and keeping cooked foods for a short period of time. Street food vendors can be used as agents for change in the behavior and practices of their clients by insisting on the latter's personal hygiene and table manners.

Local authorities are scared of the challenge by street foods demanding provision of necessary amenities and services, and leave alone the responsibility to develop the sector. The easiest alternative left to local authorities is to take immediate steps and establish policy measures that will protect the consumers. For ease of control, local authorities are advised to register all vendors, classify them where necessary and license them. This money would help upgrade hygienic standards by assisting in the provision of water and other facilities for the preparation, cooking and service of food.

One positive attitude of vendors is that they are willing to be trained in basic hygiene and sanitation, in order to produce a safer and high quality food. Vendors need to be educated through periodic exhibitions, educational talks, slides and video shows, posters and pamphlets. There is a need to ensure that by-laws on food handling, sanitation, service methods, provision of safe water, maintaining good personal hygiene and environmental sanitation are formulated and observed. Local authorities need to establish agencies for control and supervision like the Food and Drugs Department of Kampala City Council. Licensing should be considered as a means of control while regular inspection of work places and food handlers will ensure sanitation and personal hygiene practices. Health insurance seemed to be a major concern for these micro-entrepreneurs whose business relies on them alone. Credit is assumed by donor agencies to be the primary need for all micro-entrepreneurs.

Training courses should be organized for different levels of education among food handlers to increase awareness among the vendors regarding street-food related hygiene aspects. Such courses should have an established system of monitoring and evaluation to assess their effectiveness [17, 22]. It is suggested that selected members of the street food community could be trained as health workers to give necessary health messages and act as agents of change. They could receive simple certificates of attendance and be respected by their communities as links between the vendors and authorities.

Consumers themselves have an important role to play in improving street food by insisting on improved quality of food and cleanliness of the place of work. Since civil servants form a quite important category of street food consumers, consumer education should be undertaken in their work places. This should be supported by their employer, the municipal and/or national authorities in order to protect their health. In conclusion, consumers and vendors should be educated to recognize that food of better nutritional, micro-bial and chemical quality will mean better health.

Access to prize spots near cinemas or on school grounds could be granted only after the vendor has passed a course on sanitation and nutrition. Such procedures would enhance the income of vendors, improve the safety of the food sold, improve the traffic flow and appearance of downtown areas and still allow an important part of the urban food system to function well.

Acknowledgements

Thanks are due to Dr. Kamala Krishnaswami, Director, National Institute of Nutrition, Hyderabad for useful discussions.

References

1   Hansen KT: Urban women and work in Africa: A Zambian case. Transafrica Forum 1987;4:3.

2   Nelson N: How women and men get by: The sexual division of labour in the informal sector of a Nairobi squatter settlement; in Bromley R, Gerry C (eds): Causal Work and Poverty in the Third World Cities. New York, Wiley, 1979.

3   Blumberg RL: Females farming and food: Rural development and women's participation in agricultural production systems in Barbara Lewis 1981. cf Tinker I. Street Foods. Curr Sociol 1987;35: 1–110.

4   Rosette JB: Women's work in the informal sector: A Zambian case study Working Paper 3. East Lansing, Michigan State University, 1982.

5   Vercruijsse E: Fishmongers, big dealers and fishermen: Cooperation and conflict between the sexes in Ghanaian Canoe fishing; in Oppong C (ed): Female and Male in West Africa. London, Allen & Unwin, 1983.

6   Horn NE: Urban food provisioning and the role of market women in Harare, Zimbabwe. Washington, Meet Assoc Women in Development, April 15, 1987.

7   Tinker I: Street foods. Curr Sociol 1987;35:1–110.

8   Cohen M: The influence of the street food trade on women and children; in Jellife DB, Jelliffe EFP (eds): Advances in International Maternal and Child Health. Oxford, Clarendon Press, 1986, vol 6, pp 148–165.

9   CILSS: Etude du Marche Urbain Sahelien (Senegal et Haute Volta) des Céréales Locales et de Leurs Derives Susceptibles de se Subsistueter aux Importation. Paris, Macromer, 1980.

10   Atkinson SJ: Street foods; in Moleolo B (ed): Food for the Cities. Urban Nutrition Policy in Developing Countries. London, PHP Departmental Publication, London School of Hygiene and Tropical Medicine, 1992, pp 37–38.

11   Pearce TO: The place of street foods in the urban diet: A survey of Ile-Ife, Nigeria. Africa Studies Assoc Meet, Los Angeles, Department of Sociology/Anthropology University of Ife, Ile-Ife, Nigeria, 1984.

12   FAO/FBRI: Training programme for women on the safe production and sale of street foods in Nigeria. Report of the training programme held at the Conference Centre, University of Ibadan, Ibadan, 26 Nov–2 Dec, 1989. Rome, Food and Agriculture Organization of the United Nations. Ibadan, Food Basket Foundation International, 1990, pp 1–23.

13   Tinker I: The case of legalizing street foods. Ceres 1987;20:26–31.

14   Dawson RJ, Canet C: International activities in street foods. Food Control 1991;2:135–139.

15   Dawson RJ: FAO and street foods. Proc 3rd World Congr Foodborne Infections and Intoxications 16th–19th June 1992. Organised by Institute of Veterinary Medicine, Robert Von Ostertag Institute FAO/WHO Collaborative Centre for Research and Training in Food Hygiene and Zoonosis, Berlin, 1992, pp 802–805.

16   FAO: Street Foods: A summary of FAO studies and activities relating to street foods. A report, Rome, Food & Agriculture Organization, 1989, pp 1–28.

17   Nasinyama GW: Study on street foods in Kampala-Uganda. Rome, Food and Agriculture Organization Kampala, Makerere University, 1992, pp 1–37,

18   FAO: Street foods: Food and Nutrition Paper No. 46. Rome, Food & Agriculture Organization, 1990, pp 1–30.

19   Tinker I, Cohen M: Street foods as a source of income for women. Ekistics 1985;52.310:83–89.

20   Picasso E: Las Alimentadoras de Pueblo venddoas ambulantes de alimentos preparados Grupo de Trabajo; servicios urbanos Y Mujeres de Bajos Ingreos-Sumbi, Lima, Peru: SUMBI 1986; in Tinker I: Street foods. Curr Sociol 1987;35:1–110.

21   Schildkrout E: Dependence and autonomy: The economic activities of secluded Hausa women in Kano; in Oppong C (ed): Female and Male in West Africa. London, George Allen & Unwin, 1981.

22   Ashenafi M: Bacteriological profile and holding temperature of ready-to-serve food items in an open market in Awassa, Ethiopia. Trop Geo Med 1995;47:244–247.

23   EPOC: Project Notes: Street Foods. Washington, Equity Policy Centre, 1984.

24   Kujore O: Street Foods Project Proposal: A Nigerian (Ile-Ife)/EPOC proposal, 1983,

25   Cohen M. Informal Sector Activity in Regional Urban Areas: The Street Food Trade. Washington, Equity Policy Centre, 1984.

26   Posner J: Street Foods in Senegal. Equity Policy Centre, Washington, 1983.

27   Oguntona CRB, Kanye O: Contribution of street foods to nutrient intakes by Nigerian adolescents. Nutr Health 1995;10:165–171.

28   de Giusti M, de Vito E, Gisiano P, Tufi D: Hygiene standards of street foods in Benin, West Africa. Igiene Moderna 1993;99:474–481.

29   Muchnik J: Division sexuele du Travail et changement Technique: L'Artisanat Alimentaire en Republique Populaire du Benin. Int Wkshop Women's Roles in Food Self-Sufficiency and Food Strategies, Paris, January 14–19, 1985.

30   El-Sherbeeny MR, Saddik MF, Hekmat EA, Bryan FL: Microbiological profile and storage temperatures of Egyptian rice dishes. J Food Prot 1985;48:39–43.

31   Saddik MF, El-Sherbeeny MR, Bryan FL: Microbiological profiles of Egyptian raw vegetables and salads. J Food Prot 1985;48:883–886.

32   El-Sherbeeny MR, Saddik MF, Bryan FL: Microbiological profiles of foods served by street vendors in Egypt. Int J Food Microbiol 1985;2:355–364.

33   Essuman KM: Local packaging of foods in Ghana. Food Nutr Bull 1990;12:64–68.

34   Barrot P: Green packaging: Local, biodegradable and it's even edible. Ceres 1995;27:9–10.

35   Dawson RJ: International activities on street foods; in Merican Z, Ahamad N, Quee Lan Y, Moy MG, Othman NDM, Shahabudin HA, Mohamed AR (eds): Proc 1st Asian Conf Food Safety, The Challenges of the 90s, Kuala Lumpur, Sept. 2–7, 1990. Malaysia, Malaysian Institute of Food Technology, 1990, pp 129–134.

36   FAO and Department of Human Nutrition: University of Ibadan, Nigeria Report of the Study on Street Foods in Ibadan: Characteristics of Food Vendors and Consumers, Implications for Quality and Safety (FAO). Ibadan, 1987.

37   Kalpinsky R: Inappropriate products and techniques: Breakfast foods in Kenya. Rev Afr Polit Econ 1979;14:90–96.

38   Jiwa SFH, Krovacek K, Wadstrom T: Enterotoxigenic bacteria in food and water from an Ethiopian community. Appl Environ Microbiol 1981;41:1010–1019.

39   Boutrif E: Global perspectives of street foods; in Natarajan CP, Ranganna S (eds): Trends in Food Science and Technology Association of Food Science and Technologists (India). Mysore, Central Food Technological Research Institute, 1995, pp 753–759.

40   Louis ME St, Porter JD, Helal A, Drame K, Bean HN, Wells JG, Tauxe RV: Epidemic cholera in West Africa: The role of food handling and high risk foods. Am J Epidemiol 1990;131:719–728.

41   FAO and WHO: Draft Guidelines for the design of control measures for street vended foods in Africa. Joint FAO/WHO Food Standards Programme Alinorm 97/28, appendix II. Food and Agriculture Organization of the United Nations and World Health Organization, 1997, pp 17–30.

42   Anon: Food safety and tourism. Sécurité alimentarie et tourisme, Regional Conf Food and Tourism, Tunis, Nov 25–27, 1991, pp 228:93–12–C0008 Agricola data base.

Dr. Ramesh V. Bhat, National Institute of Nutrition, Indian Council of Medical Research, Jamai-Osmania P.O., Hyderabad 500 007 AP (India)
Tel. +91 40 7018909, Fax +91 40 7019074, E-Mail nin@ap.nic.in

Simopoulos AP, Bhat RV (eds): Street Foods.
World Rev Nutr Diet. Basel, Karger, 2000, vol 86, pp 123–137

....
Street Foods in Latin America

Ramesh V. Bhat, Kavita Waghray

National Institute of Nutrition, Indian Council of Medical Research,
Hyderabad, India

Latin American and Carribean countries during recent years have witnessed a deterioration in living conditions in rural areas resulting in a concomitant accelerated urbanization process. Almost 75% of the inhabitants of the hemisphere are now living in urban areas. The tremendous urban congestion especially in the capital cities forces people to travel great distances to get back to their homes. Street vending of foods which offers foodstuffs at reasonable prices makes it an ideal solution to situations stemming from the rate of growth of the cities [1]. The hectic urban life has created a steady rise in the demand for foods in the vicinity of the places of work which offer an economical tasty alternative for the people thus contributing to the proliferation of street vendors of food products. At the same time, it creates a problem of urban planners and administrators. The various national governments were concerned with the public health consequences of indiscriminate proliferation of vending of foods in the streets. Local research inputs into the various nutritional and food safety issues concerned with street foods were minimal. Considering the importance of the problem of street foods to national economy and health implications, regional studies on street foods were initiated in Columbia, Nicaragua, Guatemala, Honduras and Peru. Some of the activities include evaluating problems associated with street foods working with the governments to develop programs to improve quality and safety of foods. Studies on the socioeconomic situation including employment, improving food handling technology, training of food handlers, consumer education and the training of food inspectors and control staff (table 1).

Table 1. Projects on street foods in Latin America

Organization	Project/country
Food and Agriculture Organization (FAO)	project on street foods in Columbia, Costa Rica, Ecuador, El Salvador, Gautemala, Honduras, Nicaragua, Panama, Peru strengthen the safety and quality control of street foods in strategic areas of Bolivia socioeconomic impact of street foods in Lima
PanAmerican Health Organization (PAHO)	consumer protection with relation to possible risks associated with the consumption of street foods in Bolivia multisectorial and multidisciplinary street food control program in Bolivia project on street foods in the Dominican Republic
International Development Research Center (IDRC)	Jamaican street foods
FAO and National Authorities	design of improved technologies for preparation of street foods in Quito, Guayaquil, Cuenca Chile (project on street foods) English-speaking Carribean countries (project on street foods)

Socioeconomic Aspects

The street food industry is a part of the informal economy of the Latin American countries. However, this industry poses a variety of difficulties for the governments of the region like street food vendors invade and occupy the public spaces, contribute to the deterioration of the cities by impairing esthetics, cleanliness, traffic congestions, etc. [1].

The number of persons involved in the street food business varied from place to place. In some of the Latin American countries like the Dominican Republic, the number of people involved in the preparation/serving, etc., of street foods varied from 1 to 3 including the owner [2]. In many of the Latin American cities there are people who own a large number of street-vending establishments and they hire salaried people to operate them [1]. Not only men, women are also involved in the various activities of this informal industry. Studies conducted on street foods in a number of Latin American countries have shown an overall increase in the participation of women in the street food operation not only in the preparation and serving of foods but also in the marketing. In some countries such as Peru, Guatemala and Jamaica, about 50% of the participants in activities related to street vending of food are women while the percentage is 59% in Columbia and 64% in the rest of the South American countries [3, 4]. In some countries like Honduras, the percentage even increases up to 90% [5].

The percentage of income devoted to the purchase of street foods declines as the income of the people rises. Studies carried out in Latin American countries like Peru have shown that the consumers spend a considerable portion of their overall budget on street foods [4]. As much as 20–30% of the food budget of urban families is spent on street foods [5].

In some of the Latin American countries like Jamaica the cost of the street foods was based on its nutrient content. Powell et al. [3] reported that when energy and protein supplied by a dollar worth of each item is compared, most foods in the commercially prepared solids groups gave the best value for money. Foods with best cost nutrient values are button cookies, water crackers, jackass corn and homemade asham. When energy is the criterion, the 6 best buys in descending order are button cookies, asham, home-made banana chips, water crackers, rough drop cookies and jackass corn (407–910 kcal per 1 $). Unlike for proteins the best buys in descending order are button cookies, water crackers, asham and cheese buns (8–10 g per 1 $). Liquids whether homemade or commercially processed provided low amounts of energy and protein per dollar.

In Bolivia, a traditional meal providing 568 kcal costs $0.50, while in Ecuador, meals like meat with potatoes, chicken and meat, and fish with rice cost $0.50, $0.60, and $0.60, respectively [6].

Profile of Street Food Vendors

The number of street food vendors varied in the different Latin American countries depending upon the population and the role of urbanization. Different studies conducted in Latin America revealed that there is wide variation in the age of the vendors. Studies conducted by FAO [4] in Peru revealed that the majority of the vendors were 21–45 years old. Unlike in Jamaica the age of vendors ranged from 14 to 78 years with a mean age of 35.5 years, the female vendors being older than their male counterparts [3].

In the Latin American countries, the level of formal education for the street food vendors is rather low with most of them having received less than 8 years of formal schooling [4]. The illiteracy rate of street food vendors in some of the Latin American countries such as Peru (11.5%) is considered high. In Ecuador, 54% had received a primary education with the remainder being less educated. While in Columbia 56% of the vendors had received elementary school education and 17% some secondary school education. Unlike in Jamaica where 70% of the 300 street food vendors interviewed had higher than primary level education [5]. There was no correlation between the level of income and educational background of the street vendors.

Studies conducted by FAO [4] in Latin American countries like Columbia, Ecuador, Peru, etc., have shown that most of the street food vendors earn more than the country's minimum wage [1]. In Ecuador, 68% of the street food vendors were making equivalent to or more than the minimum wage [7].

Personal hygiene among the street food vendors varied. In Peru, 76% of the vendors did not meet the national standards set for clean clothes even though 52% of them wore coverings over their clothes. Of those wearing coverings 74% were female and 26% were male. Even in Columbia 56% of the vendors wore coverings over their regular street clothes.

The level of formal education may be a contributing factor to the general lack of knowledge of hygiene and food sanitation among the street food vendors. The Peruvian study showed that the higher the educational level of the vendors, the better the hygienic practices. In general, women pursued better general hygienic practices than men [8].

Profile of Consumers

There was a wide variation among the age group and educational level of the consumers who consumed street foods. Specific studies to substantiate the data are not available.

In Jamaica, the consumers were mainly workforce like female factory workers, construction workers, schoolchildren (primary and higher schoolchildren of both sexes) [3].

Street foods play an important role in diets of people, especially the urban poor, residing in Latin American countries. Street foods contribute up to 35% of a given individual's daily food intake [9]. Webb and Hyatt [10] reported that 18% of the Carribean recommended dietary allowance of energy and 25% of actual average daily intake of food for the secondary schoolchildren in Haiti was provided by street food alone. In Jamaica 10–30% of the daily requirements of energy and protein in school population were provided by some selected street foods like sandwiches, cheese buns, biscuits and cookies, and chocolate/peanut candy bars. Milk-based beverages, fruits, corn snacks and nonmilk beverages provided less than 10% of their requirements for energy and protein. Prepared traditional homemade meals sold by vendors such as jerked chicken and bread provided over 100% of the daily protein requirements for adult females and just that percentage for the adult male construction worker. Their energy contribution ranged from 23.0 to 7.5% for these two consumer groups, respectively. The energy and protein contributions of soups are considerably less than jerked chicken contributing 13.7–9.9% energy and 25.7–14.9% protein for adults, while cheese buns, biscuits and cookies make a significant contribution to both their energy and protein intake [3]. In Ecuador, the percentage of energy requirements provided by meals like meat with potatoes is 14% of the total daily requirement, chicken and meat (29%), and fish with rice (40%) [6].

In no study was it shown consumers chose a particular food for its nutritional value. In Honduras, the taste of the food was the primary reason for selection. Generally, the next most popular reasons for selecting street foods were their low cost followed by their convenience/availability [5]. As elsewhere in the world urban schoolchildren have been identified as significant purchasers of street foods in Latin American countries such as Haiti [9]. This is readily apparent as vendors congregate in front of schools to sell their products to students of all ages [10].

Profile of Street Foods Sold

A variety of street foods are sold in different Latin American countries. However, their number varied from country to country ranging from 3 varieties in Peru, 9 in Trinidad, 16 in the Dominican Republic and as many as 20 varieties in Jamaica. The different types of food varied from snack preparations, sweet meats, beverages (hot and cold) to full course meals (table 2).

The different raw materials required by the street food vendors for the preparation of food were procured from wholesale outlets and municipal market on cash payment in Jamaica [3]. This practice varied from place to place in other Latin American countries depending upon the vendors' financial situation.

Fuel used by the street food vendors for the preparation of street foods varied from place to place depending upon the availability and cost of the resources. In Haiti, street food vendors used small metal charcoal stoves [10]. Similar observations were also made in the Dominican Republic. The vendors cooked the food over charcoal in a metal tire rim (supported by three legs welded to the rim) [2]. Place of preparation of the street foods varied depending upon the convenience of the vendor. Bryan et al. [2] reported that the street food vendors in the Dominican Republic prepared the food near the site in the early hours and later served by reheating on demand. While some of the vendors prepared few items at home at night and served it on the same or the next day.

Table 2. Profile of street foods sold in Latin America

Country	Street food dishes	Ref. No.
Bolivia	soaked boiled and watered lupines	11
Dominican Republic	fried cheese, plantains, fried corn, bollito, fried wheat torreja, boiled and deep-fried yuca beef stew, moro chicken, meat, bacito, fried chicken, chicharron fried, ham, pieces of fried pig's head, chuleta, fried sausage, fried beef, fresh cheese, moro rice, beans, pastel de hoja	2
Jamaica	jerked chicken and bread, peppered shrimps, Irish moss with milk, stewed chicken, tamarind syrup, stewed beef, magnum force, fish, tea, cow's skin soup, Irish moss without milk, carbonated soft drinks, sky juice. Heineken beer, red stripe beer, fruit-flavored drink, boxed milk, fresh juices, orange, sugar cane, black mango, homemade banana chips, button cookies, corned beef sandwich, ginger log bun, water crackers, coconut crunch cookies, animal-shaped crackers, golden crackers, corn/sugar snacks, cheese twist, jackass corn, rough drop cookies, asham, tamarind balls, chocolate/peanut bar (catch), ice cream cones	3
Peru	fried fish, ceviche, beef hearts, soaked boiled and watered lupines	2, 11, 12
Trinidad	black pudding, doubles, roti (dhal pourie), mango chutney, punch drinks, seamoss, local sweets, preserved fruits, ice creams	13

A wide range of processing methods were used by the street food vendors in the preparation of street foods. Only few studies have discussed the different types of methods used by the vendors for preparation of street foods. Street food vendors in Haiti prepared the different types of foods by boiling, frying, roasting, or home baking (traditional baking). Beverages were prepared by boiling, juicing and fermenting [10]. In the Dominican Republic various types of foods were prepared by vendors by boiling, deep-fat frying and soaking. Different street food vendors in Trinidad prepared the food using a roti cooker and different methods like boiling, frying, marinating and cooking [2].

The different containers/materials used by the street food vendors for storage and display of street food varied in Latin American countries. In Haiti, the foods were stored and displayed in several types of containers like flat, shallow and round woven trays, shallow rectangular metal bins, wooden trays, baskets, metal pots, bowls (plastic, metal) and portable wooden boxes that open up. For display tables, wheel barrows, portable carts on wheels, coolers, bottles, and clothes laid on ground were used [14]. In Peru portable water was frequently stored in uncovered old containers which are not easy to wash [5]. While in the Dominican Republic the cooked foods were stored/displayed by the vendors in pots, cabinets of the stand, on top of cabinet in a white metal pan, on white paper in shelves, and glass-encased cabinets with several light bulbs (located inside to provide illumination and to generate heat) [2].

The serving containers used by the street food vendors in different parts of Latin America were based on their traditions. Some of the vendors in the Dominican Republic used large metal spoons for serving. The general practice followed by vendors in different parts of the world of providing serving containers to the customers was not observed by some vendors in the Dominican Republic. Unlike here in few cases the customers brought their own eating utensils like plates, bowls or pots [2].

In some Latin American countries like Peru, the sanitary conditions of the utensils and tableware were judged substandard in 76–89% of the inspection [5]. A variety of packaging material were used by the street food vendors in Latin America. In Jamaica vendors used aluminum foil, cellophane/plastic bags, newsprint/wax wrapping papers, cardboard lunch boxes, plastic ice cream containers and glass bottles [3]. Vendors in Haiti used paper such as newsprint as the main packaging material [10] while in the Dominican Republic vendors used banana leaves for packaging [2].

Use of leftover food items varied from vendor to vendor. In the Dominican Republic some of the vendors carried the leftover food home and stored it in a refrigerator, while others piled the food into a plastic bucket and kept it in the cabinet overnight and served the same cold food the next day. They heated the food if customers demanded or else served it at room temperature [2].

Among the most critical problems observed in the various studies in Latin America was lack of an adequate supply of potable water for cooking, washing, cooking utensils covers, preparing ice, beverages, drinking and personal hygiene [4]. In Peru, 94% of the vendors used public portable water in their food business and the rest of them obtained water from van tanks in the suburban areas [8]. In Columbia, it was shown that 98% of the street vendors were without any system for supply of good quality water, in sufficient quantity. This situation is similar in other countries and compels the vendors to use the same water repeatedly without changing it even a single time during the day. Such a practice leads to the water becoming a focus for the growth of bacteria from high levels of dissolved organic matter. If contaminated with pathogenic bacteria like *Salmonella, Shigella, Yersinia*, and *Staphylococcus aureus,* the water can pose a serious health hazard [1, 15, 16].

Similar situations were also observed in the Dominican Republic. Running water was seldom available at the stands. Hand, dish and utensil washing was usually done in one or more buckets or pans of water (sometimes without soap) and disinfection was rarely done [2].

Disposal of waste water and garbage was shown to be a major problem in Latin American countries. This is a universal problem applicable to all the countries in the world. In Lima, Peru, 70% of the garbage was collected and disposed of by the municipalities but 30% of the garbage as well as nearly 40% of the waste water was disposed of in the streets encouraging rodents and the proliferation of mosquitoes and flies thus causing a sanitation problem [6]. In addition, the absence of sanitary facilities (toilet) within reach of the vendors forces them to excrete their body wastes in the vicinity or nearby secluded areas without properly washing their hands afterwards. The situations described are typical of street vending in many places throughout the world as well as in the Dominican Republic [2].

Like in other parts of the world even in Latin American countries street food vendors were located in areas where people congregate in large numbers. Underwood [14] reported that roadside selling of cooked foods and beverages by the vendors was observed daily throughout Haiti. Similar observations were also made by Webb and Hyatt [10] in Haiti. They reported that vendors were most frequently seen along the sidewalks of major streets, or grouped together at the corners. The density of the vendors was near shopping areas and markets, schools, public transportation stations, cinemas, tourist attractions, and a few were also seen in residential areas. Ambulatory vendors were also found to follow set routes calling out their wares as they travelled to alert potential customers to their presence in the neighborhood. In other Latin American countries such as the Dominican Republic, the street vendors were seen near work places, markets, schools, parks, recreation events (places), and bus stops as large crowds of people congregated in these locations [2].

There was a wide variation in the type of vending vehicles used by the street vendors in the Latin American countries. In Peru fresh fish fry was prepared on portable stoves and sold on busy street corners. And almost everywhere women sold nuts from baskets which they carried on their heads. Along with this the vendors also sold soups and meals to the customers from street stalls located under a cloth shade held up by poles or matting [12]. In Jamaica, 88% of the vendors out of 300 were stationary, especially at sites where sales tended to be good, and the rest were mobile [3]. Bryan et al [2] reported that in the Dominican Republic the street vendors used different types of vending vehicles. Some of them were stationary and had rectangular (cart), wooden stands under the shade of a tree and some had properly constructed places.

Information regarding the material used in the construction of vending vehicles in Latin America is meager. Mostly, it depends on the location of the vending site. Bryan et al. [2] reported in the Dominican Republic that stands and carts used by the street food vendors are often crudely constructed. The construction materials used by them included metal frames, plastic sheets and wood.

Quality of Street Food in Latin America

Several studies have been conducted in Latin America on quality aspects of street foods including that of nutritional, chemical and microbial quality, presence of food additives, and contaminants. However, exclusive studies on physical quality such as the presence of dirt, filth and insect excreta are meager [5]. According to Bryan et al. [2] though attempts were made to protect food from flies in the Dominican Republic they were ineffective. Arambulo et al. [1] reported that in Latin American countries substances such as nitrites and nitrates, unauthorized coloring agents, preservatives like benzoates, sorbates and metabisulfites, texturizers and sweeteners were used widely. These substances can be assumed to have contributed to the epidemiologic transition in the morbidity and mortality structure of the countries where chronic diseases, as well as cancer, are becoming more and more frequent. The risks include poisonous substances such as lead residues (from automobile exhausts), pesticide residues in fruit and vegetables and poisonous substances originating during food preparation and processing [1].

Nutritional Value
The nutritional value of the foods sold in Latin American countries varied from place to place and vendor to vendor depending on the tradition, culture and raw materials used. For example, in Jamaica the energy contribution of street foods which were commercially prepared solids ranged from 317 to 611 kcal/ 100 g. There was a wide variation in energy contribution of traditional home-made solids and liquids ranging from 40 kcal/100 g in soups to 496 kcal/100 g in banana chips. The energy value of commercially prepared liquids except for ice cream cones and natural foods were generally low, i.e. 11–65 kcal/ 100 g. Protein content varied widely ranging from 1.1 to 20.7 g in most of the foods and was minimal in the natural foods and commercial fruit-flavored beverages [3]. In Bolivia, a traditional meal sold by the street food vendor provides 568 kcal [6].

Microbial Contamination
Studies conducted in Latin American countries have confirmed the presence of microbial contamination in the food sold by the street food vendors.

A study conducted in Bolivia in 1985, revealed that 30% of 152 samples showed the presence of *E. coli, Salmonella* sp. and *S. aureus*.

A later study carried out during 1987–1989 revealed that 14% of 565 samples of street foods were contaminated with *E. coli* and 51% of products had a level of mesophillic aerobic microorganisms above the safe level (10^4/g) [6]. Studies carried out in Ecuador in 1990 showed that 76.5% of the street food samples (n = 250) were contaminated with *S. aureus* and other microorganisms [6]. In Peru, studies conducted revealed the presence of *S. aureus* in the 'ceviche' (a dish prepared with fresh fish and cheese). Actually, the fresh cheese showed the presence of *S. aureus* [6]. Studies carried out in other Latin American countries like El Salvador, Guatemala, Honduras, and Nicaragua from 1982 to 1990 showed that more than 50% of the samples were contaminated according to microbiological national criteria. Exact comparison of the results may not be possible due to the differences among types of samples analyzed and criteria used to quantify them as 'contaminated'. It is evident from these studies that the risk of transmission of foodborne diseases is certainly a reality [6].

Though such studies on microbial contamination of street-vended foods in Honduras have been conducted earlier too, the cholera epidemic in Latin America in the early 1990s provided an impetus for microbiological surveillance activities. Despite these, no standards have been established for street foods. General prevention and control activities were carried out by the various institutions involved, primarily the Ministry of Public Health and the Ministry of Natural Resources. Microorganism control in Honduras includes coliform bacteria (*E. coli*) total bacterial count, *S. aureus, Vibrio cholerae, Parahemolytic vibrio, Salmonella*, fungi and yeasts [17].

Among the different snack preparation like doubles, roti, chutney, and black pudding sold by the street food vendors in Trinidad, black pudding was significantly more contaminated with *S. aureus* (73%). It also yielded 10 strains of *Salmonella* and 42.3% of the samples showed the presence of *E. coli*. This preparation, i.e. black pudding posed a greater health risk to the consumers. Some roti samples also revealed the presence of *S. aureus* (24%) and *E. coli* (20%) [13]. Food preparations such as bacito (fried fish), fried chicken, fried pig's head pieces, fried ham, chicharron (fried pork with rind attached), corn bollito, wheat torreja, sausage, beef, ham, (chuleta) pork belly, chicharron (grilled pork ribs) and fresh cheese, sold by the street food vendors in the Dominican Republic showed the presence of high levels of AMCC/g after leaving overnight for 1 or 2 days (1.3×10^3–1.4×10^9/g) and the level reduced on reheating the products. Some of these products like chicken, pig's head pieces, ham, chicharron, sausage, and beef, which were deep fried, also showed the presence of *Clostridium perfringens* ranging from

<10 to 5.0×10^2/g. Pastel de hoja (minced meat in mashed plantains wrapped in banana leaves) had an AMCC of 1.0×10^5/g and *B. cereus* count of 1.5×10^3/g [2].

Ice creams sold by vendors in Trinidad were of poor bacterial quality. Adesiyun [13] reported that 18 (27.3%) of 66 ice cream samples were positive for *S. aureus* and 2 (3.0%) were positive for *E. coli*. Of 26 snow cone samples 2 (7.7%) had *S. aureus* and 2 (7.7%) had *E. coli* contamination. Studies conducted by major University of San Marcos on street foods revealed the presence of *V. cholerae* in ice creams [6]. The other dairy products such as local milk-based sweets (1 of 29 samples), punch drinks (11.1% of 18) showed the presence of *S. aureus*. Seamoss samples (33.3% of 15 samples) were contaminated with *E. coli* [13].

In the Dominican Republic concentrated milk and orange juice sold by vendors had an AMCC of 2.7×10^6/g [2]. The sweet meats like preserved fruits (mangoes, plumbs and cherries) and local sweets (milk-based preparations) sold by the street vendors in sale outlets in Trinidad also revealed the presence of *S. aureus* in 3.4% of 29 samples [13].

The samples of full-course meal foods like beans, rice moro (rice and bean preparation), chicken, and meat sold by the street vendors in the Dominican Republic showed the presence of aerobic mesophillic colony counts (AMCC)/g ranging from 5.0×10^2 to 1.8×10^8. Bean samples also showed the presence of *B. cereus* and *C. perfringens* <10/g. While the rice samples also contained *B. cereus* 1.0×10^3/g. The moro samples also showed the presence of *B. cereus* 2×10^2/g. Chicken and meat samples showed the presence of *C. perfringens* <10/g [2].

The water samples collected from the street vendors in the Dominican Republic showed the presence of aerophillic mesophillic colony counts ranging from 1.5×10^3 to 9×10^3/ml, *E. coli* >10 ml [2].

Hazard analysis was carried out in the Dominican Republic of different foods such as fried chicken, fried pork ribs with rind, fried fish, fried ham and pieces of fried pig's head, pork belly, ham, beef, sausage, cheese, plantains, corn bollito (corn dough with anise), wheat torreja (containing salted fish, green pepper and vegetables) and boiled yuca sold by street vendors at four street-vending stands. The results revealed that the problem was keeping cooked foods at ambient temperature for 13 h or longer. Low counts of *B. cereus* and *C. perfringens* were observed which might be due to a low a_w at the surface of fried foods [2].

In countries where street-vended foods is common there is usually a lack of information about the incidence of foodborne diseases and investigations of outbreaks of these diseases is seldom done. Yet diarrheal diseases are commonly experienced by persons of all ages. The relative importance of street-vended foods in contributing to diarrheal diseases in general and outbreaks of foodborne diseases in particular is undefined [2]. In Peru, the cases of food-borne diseases 'reported' from 1985 to 1988 were 35,000/year (on an average) with a rate of 2,200 cases/100,000 inhabitants. During the cholera epidemic which affected the country in 1991, a case study conducted in Piura (between February-March 1991) on 50 cases and 100 controls showed a significant relationship between the presence of illness and the consumption of beverages and foods sold in the streets [6].

Regulation of Street Foods

The regulation of street foods in Latin American countries varied from country to country. In Venezuela, the sale of street foods is regulated by a ministerial resolution: G-375 of March 5, 1990 [17]. Bolivia has a specific multisectorial and multidisciplinary street food control program with involve-ment of the Ministry of Social Welfare and Public Health, the Mayors' Officers and the Ministry of Education. With the appearance of the cholera epidemic, this program on contamination control was introduced for food handlers particularly for short-stemmed vegetables and for produce irrigated with con-taminated water [17].

There is a law in the Dominican Republic that prohibits vending on streets, but it is not enforced [19]. In Peru, Ministerial Resolution No. 0014-92-SA/DM of January 17, 1992, which repeals the Resolution of the Deputy Minister of Health No. 103–87-SA of August 18, 1987, hygiene rules governing the sale of foods on public thoroughfares have been promulgated. They cover: (i) health and hygiene standards to be observed in the preparation and sale of foods and beverages on public thoroughfares; (ii) rules to ensure that foods or beverages are fit for human consumption; (iii) hygiene requirements relating to food handlers/vendors, sales points, and to preparation, storage and serving of foods; (iv) registration and control, and sanctions [20].

In Ecuador and Columbia, 30 and 20% of the vendors had a vending license and 63 and 10% had a health certificate. In Peru, only 42% of the vendors had undergone a medical examination and carried a health certificate. In Guatemala, 2,500 street food vendors were licensed while 7,500 were not [4]. In Barbados, control on food vendors needed to be reinforced which was being done partly through education [17].

In Paraguay, CONAPRA 1992 implemented an action plan called the Emergency Plan for Microbiological Control in food. In this program street foods were also included [17].

The main problems Honduras has encountered in implementing programs to prevent and/or control microbiological contamination in food are the lack of interagency coordinating mechanisms, the scarcity of qualified and/or specialized staff, the lack of standardized norms, the low level of awareness in the public and private sectors and the lack of epidemiological surveillance system for foodborne disease [17].

At one time when the law was strictly enforced by authorities in the Dominican Republic, street-vending operations were closed and unsanitary equipment was destroyed. Vending operations however, were reestablished within a short time. This was so because the general public accepted street-vending practices such as holding cooked food for several hours at ambient (room) temperature. The situation in many food service establishments and in many homes did not differ greatly from those used by the vendors. Furthermore, some vending (like sale of packaged low moisture food) operations were basically safe.

The Codex coordinating committee for Latin America and the Caribbean islands at its 5th session 1987 proposed a preliminary draft code [5].

Suggestions for Improvement of Street Foods in Latin America

Bryan et al. [2] reported that in the Dominican Republic enforcement of the law banning street vendors did not work in the past mainly due to lack of understanding of hazards and safe practices. The remedy, suggested to reach the core of the problem is education of public health personnel, educating of street vendors and food service personnel and education of the public who either purchase street-vended foods or become vendors themselves. Street vendors will need to be trained either in courses or during visits to their facilities. This will be challenging because of the transient nature of some vendors, their long hours of operation, and the limited financial resources available to make some of the changes needed in their operations to ensure the safety of food. Developing training in cooperation with vending trade associations, where they exist will facilitate this endeavor and stimulate action. Illustrated leaflets showing acceptable practices could be pasted at the stands or on carts or nearby for both vendor and purchaser of vended food to see and heed [21].

In studies conducted in Peru and Columbia, it has been shown that the street food vendors are willing to accept training in basic hygiene and sanitation in order to produce safe and better foods [4]. In Peru and Columbia, training materials have been designed and used in training with local authorities. However, only a few Latin American countries have been involved in training programs and much remains to be done.

Consumer education is necessary in order to enable them to evaluate the nutrition and safety value of street foods. Consumers must be able to protect themselves from possible health hazards. Priorities in consumer protection and education should be directed towards all ages of people but particularly towards schoolchildren [4, 21].

Prospective consumers of street-vended foods should be alerted to the hazards and cautioned to request that the cooked foods they select be reheated (fried) before they purchase them. Use of various mass media – television, radio, newspaper – has been considered to transmit the message. If practical, educational endeavors should be coordinated between official monitoring agencies, public education departments, and consumer groups. Education in food safety also needs to be incorporated into health education programs in school because the pupils either are or will become customers of street vendors in the near future and some may become vendors themselves. Appropriate health education materials must be developed from use by teachers and no doubt teachers will have to be trained in the principles of food safety as well as in the use of the materials [2].

Training programs for the public health personnel should be conducted. Different aspects like microbiological hazards and their solutions, food processing preparation technology, critical control points, practical control measures and monitoring procedures, principles of food microbiology and food safety need to be incorporated. Limitations of current practices, emphasizing microbiological hazards and not aesthetics, dispel defensive reactions, teach the new approach and stimulate trainees to take actions should also be discussed. To achieve this, program resources and priorities should be shifted away from such practices as health certificates for food workers and expiry dates on packages (for example) to solutions of time, temperature and contamination hazards. As codes of practices or guidelines are developed, CCP criteria for satisfactory practices, monitoring procedures and actions to be taken when CCP are out of control should also be specified. Foodborne disease surveillance data should be sought and used to give direction to food safety activity [2].

Acknowledgment

Thanks are due to Dr. Kamala Krishnaswami, Director, National Institute of Nutrition, Hyderabad for useful discussion.

References

1   Arambulo P III, Cuellar J, Estupinan J, Ruiz A: Street foods: A Latin American perspective; in Natarjan CP, Ranganna S (eds): Trends in Food Science and Technology. Mysore, Association of Food Science and Technologists (India) Central Food Technological Research Institute, 1995, pp 760–770.
2   Bryan FL, Michanie SC, Alvarez P, Paniague A: Critical control points of street vended foods in the Dominican Republic. J Food Prot 1988;51:373–378.
3   Powell D, Wint E, Brodber E, Campbell V: The Jamaican street food study. Cajanus 1989;22:13–36.
4   FAO: A Summary of FAO Studies and Other Activities Relating to Street Foods, Rome, FAO (of the United Nations), 1989.
5   FAO: Street Foods. FAO Food and Nutrition Paper No 46. Rome, FAO, 1990, pp 1–24.
6   Randell AW, Gonzalez MLC, Dawson RJ: FAO Activities in Latin America and the Caribbean to Control the Spread of Cholera. Rome, FAO, 1992, pp 1–10.
7   Dawson RJ, Canet C: International activities in street foods. Food Control 1991;2:135–139.
8   Dawson RJ: International activities on street foods. Proc 1st Asian Conf Food Safety the Challenges of the 90s. Kuala Lumpur, Sept 2–7, 1990, pp 129–134.
9   EPOC: EPOC Project Notes: Street Foods. Washington, Equity Policy Center, 1984.
10 Webb RE, Hyatt SA: Haitian street foods and their nutritional contribution to dietary intake. Ecol Food Nutr 1988;21:199–209.
11 Cremer HD: Current aspects on legumes as a food constituent in Latin America with special emphasis on lupines: Introduction. Qual Plant Foods Hum Nutr 1983;32:95–100.
12 Tinker I: The case of legalizing street foods. Ceres, FAO Rev 1987;20:26–31.
13 Adesiyun AA: Bacteriologic quality of some Trinidadian ready-to-consume foods and drinks and possible health risks to consumers. J Food Prot 1995;58:651–655.
14 Underwood FW: The marketing system in Peasant Haiti. Yale University Publications in Anthropology, No 60 (reprint). New Haven, HRAF Press, 1970.
15 FAO and PAHO: Informe del Taller FAO/OPS Latino americano sobre Alimentos Vendidos en la Via Publica 21–25 Octubre 1985, Lima Peru. Washington, Pan American Health Organization, 1985.
16 Boutrif E: Global perspectives of street foods; in Natarjan CP, Ranganna S (eds): Trends in Food Science and Technology. Mysore, Association of Food Science and Technologists (India), Central Food Technological Research Institute, 1995, pp 753–759.
17 FAO and PAHO: Joint FAO/PAHO Regional Workshop on Microbiological Contamination of Foods and its Implication for International Trade. Rome, FAO, 1993, pp 1–29.
18 Randell AW, Gonzalez MLC, Dawson RJ: FAO activities in Latin America and the Caribbean to control the spread of cholera; in Pestane de Castro AF, Alemieda WF (eds): Cholera on the American Continent. Washington, ILSI Press, 1993, pp 98–106.
19 Bernabel G: Higiene y control de Calidad de alimentos vendidos en via publica. Taller Latinoamericano FAO/OPS sobre alimentos comercializados in la Via Publica Lima Peru. HPV/FOS/0311V/111/86. Washington, Pan American Health Organization, 1985.
20 Arambulo P III, Almeida CR, Cuellar SJ, Beelotlo AJ: Street food vending in Latin America. Bull Pan Am Hlth Org 1994;28:344–354.
21 Anon: Sale of foods – Peru. Int Dig Hlth Legis 1994;45:346.

Dr. Ramesh V. Bhat, National Institute of Nutrition, Indian Council of Medical Research, Jamai-Osmania P.O., Hyderabad 500 007 AP (India)
Tel. +91 40 7018909, Fax +91 40 7019074, E-Mail nin@ap.nic.in

Simopoulos AP, Bhat RV (eds): Street Foods.
World Rev Nutr Diet. Basel, Karger, 2000, vol 86, pp 138–154

....

Sale of Street Food in Latin America

The Mexican Case: Joy or Jeopardy?

Miriam Muñoz de Chávez, Adolfo Chávez Villasana,
Miram Chávez Muñoz, Igor Eichin Vuskovic

National Cancer Institute, National Nutrition Institute 'S.Z.', National School of
Anthropology and History, Metropolitan University, Xochimilco, Mexico

Have you ever visited a public market in Mexico, Guatemala, Panama, Colombia, Venezuela, Peru or Brazil? Have you ever stopped to eat delicious Mayan-style pork tacos, turnovers filled with corn fungus or squash flower, octopus stuffed crepes, crab, cassava, 'alcapurrias' or grasshoppers with lime juice and chili, agave worms or a 'come back to life' seafood cocktail? If you have not, you have been missing a large part of the Mexican, Guatemalan, Panamanian, Colombian, Venezuelan, Peruvian and Brazilian folklore, taste, smell and color. And if you have visited these countries, it will be easier for you to understand the information in this chapter.

In Latin America, the demand for eating out is proportional to the size and complexity of a city. In small villages, schoolchildren like and probably need treats [1], and a few adult males go out to chat, have a drink and eat snacks. However, the mass sale of street food only occurs in major cities and has dramatically increased in the last 20 years.

Governments dislike the sale of street foods, mainly because it is not easy to collect taxes or to control the flow of food, public health and nutritional quality. The sale of street food is one of the bases of the so-called 'underground economy' and perhaps the most difficult to control and regulate [2]. It has a definite social value, which is to provide food to an important part of society, i.e. low-income employees and workers who must eat something to continue working. This need for eating in the street is associated with many changes in modern urban societies in Latin America: growing job access for women, the need to hold several jobs, the difficulties involved in preparing and even purchasing traditional food, together with advertising and many other economic and cultural factors [3].

The situation of Mexico City will be discussed because it is the one most directly familiar to us. Mexico City is an example of a Latin American city whose inhabitants are within a medium income range of about USD 4,000 per person per year, which is not any different from other Latin American cities. In addition, there are serious problems such as size and socioeconomic inequality according to sectors and neighborhoods. These two phenomena occur in many other cities such as Sao Paolo, Caracas, or Guatemala City to a greater or lesser extent.

Mexico City has another feature characteristic of the Mesoamerican region: 'tacos'. 'Tacos' are flat round corn tortillas, the size of the palm of the hand or a little bit larger, with food placed in the middle. They are rolled with a certain technique and eaten without the need for a plate or a fork. It is quite likely that 20 or 30 million of these corn tortilla rolls are sold per day in the city's metropolitan area, since over half of the city's street food is sold in this inexpensive and easy way [4, 5].

History of Street Vendors

The tradition of selling food in the streets dates back to pre-Hispanic times (fig. 1). The Museum of Anthropology in Mexico City shows a model of a market according to the stories told by the first historians to arrive with the Spanish conquerors. There was a wide variety of foods. Activities undertaken in markets that are currently called by their original name 'tianguis' were confined to bartering foods, basically those originating in the fertile lake surrounding the city, and of the floating gardens of 'chinanpas' and others of different regions. Cacao beans were very valuable and were used as currency, showing not only the liking for this commodity, but also its high value in the marketplace. Other products included amaranth, various species of tomatoes, wild greens or 'quelites', and many fruits; and animals to eat such as turkey and the native dogs called 'escuincles' [6].

Even then, corn was the most important commodity and there were varieties of different colors. Descriptions only mention the sale of ready-made 'tortillas', and it is possible that during the business hours some beverages such as 'aguamiel' (a sweet natural agave juice), 'pulque' (a fermented agave juice), 'tepache' (a fermented beverage made from pineapple) and perhaps others were sold.

The impact of the Spanish conquest put an end to all these activities that were very important in the life and development of the population. As a result

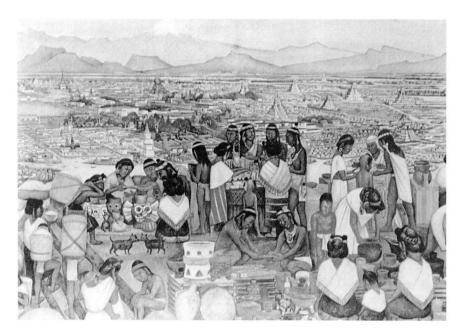

Fig. 1. Street market in pre-Hispanic times.

of famines and epidemics, the population dropped from 12.5 to 1.5 million [7]. Agriculture was almost restricted to growing basic commodities: corn, beans, and chilies. At that time, animal food was limited to the elite, the powerful members of the city. This situation continued from the 17th to the 19th century, when several foods from Europe and many from Asia arrived in the 'Nao de China' (a galleon from the Philippines), so major food trade began little by little, to such a degree that Mexico became a true worldwide food 'crossroad'. Mexico contributed important foods such as corn, beans, chilies, cacao and tomatoes. Peru contributed potatoes and Latin America as a whole contributed a huge wealth of roots, fruits and vegetables. Both in Mexico and in the other countries of the Americas, markets and foods diversified, benefitting mainly the privileged classes, because in rural areas food continued to be scarce and monotonous.

With time cities grew gradually, and after independence in 1821 the basic Mexican diet was established. This diet was very different for the poor; only corn tortillas, beans and chilies, either alone or in a tomato sauce, 'pulque' (a fermented milky beverage from various species of agave), and a few vegetables. The affluent ate meat and stew and 'moles' (a Mexican hot sauce of chilies, other spices and sometimes chocolate served with various meats). An important feature was that during the 18th and 19th centuries door-to-door sale of products greatly developed. The rich did not have to go to market: street vendors constantly passed by shouting the products for sale in different voices and tones. This still occurred in the first half of the 20th century [8].

Culture, Physiology, and Street Food

To a certain degree street food is at the same time the joy and jeopardy of Mexicans. 'Joy', because it means they can eat deliciously, according to their culture, and 'jeopardy' because it is not always nutritious and may increase the risk for infections and above all for a wide range of chronic diseases. The most sold items are closely related to culture and traditions. People relate them to life and death, health and sickness, sadness and joy, and pleasure and suffering. They are tasty, inexpensive, readily available, and frequently provide the lower classes with a large amount of high-quality animal protein, such as pork, mutton and beef, and even omega-3 fatty acids from several seafoods and certain fish. They also provide antioxidants and phytochemicals in fruit and fruit juices, such as prickly pear, pineapple, orange and yam bean; and vegetable juices, such as nopal pads, tomato, cucumber, beet, celery and alfalfa. All this, in addition to the energy, fiber and calcium contained in tortillas.

It is likely that the Mexican population at large, basically those who have Indoamerican genes (accounting for over 60%) [9] are prone to various chronic and degenerative conditions (mainly those linked to insulin resistance and obesity), such as diabetes, high blood pressure, atherosclerosis and cancer. In the early stages of life, the individual's metabolic demands are adapted to the 'thrifty gene', when energy consumption does not go beyond certain levels and physical activity is considerable. With age and increased consumption of foods high in calories and saturated fatty acids, when protective bioactive phytochemicals are lacking and physical activity is decreased, the whole metabolism is affected and it is not known whether it is diet, particularly lipids, or obesity, or the genes that may lead to the insulin resistance syndrome and to the above chronic conditions and the early aging process. The fact is, there is a clear relationship between the type and amount of street food consumed, particularly fatty, fried tacos made with animal products often much adulterated and the prevalence of chronic diseases [10].

It is also customary to associate street food with another very common phenomenon, the fact that that the harm comes from the bacterial contamination of the products on sale that are almost always exposed to dust, high temperatures, and carelessly washed food or hands, leading to several types of communicable diseases, mainly gastrointestinal disorders. Street food is well

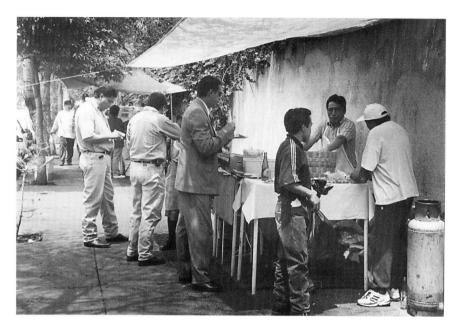

Fig. 2. Typical street vendor selling tacos.

known for its high degree of contamination; however, the little quantified information available, such as epidemic outbreaks, shows that paradoxically the incidence of acute diarrheic diseases is very low, particularly if compared with the theoretical risk of contamination. Many foods are prepared in low-income households one day before, are left overnight without refrigeration and are sold the next day. In theory, this should give rise to many problems. Unfortunately, there are no statistics about the number of cases actually caused by the intake of street food, although data on absenteeism in various work centers are available, which show that the problem may be significant [11].

Is there a gene similar to the 'thrifty gene' associated with obesity that leads to chronic conditions whose effect is to protect malnourished populations from the attack of several organisms? Could it simply be the result of immunity to household bacteria caused by repeated exposure? It is known that the famous 'Montezuma's revenge' occurs frequently in visitors from other cities and especially from abroad. They often get sick and at times very seriously ill.

It is likely that in Mexico City over five million people eat out 5 business days a week, and a modest estimate suggests that at least 20–30 million 'tacos' are sold in the street stalls per day (fig. 2). It is important to bear in mind that there are people eating street food 24 h a day and two or more tacos each time. There are 'rush hours' basically at noon, which is 'snack time', meaning that those people get home to have lunch at 3 or 4 in the afternoon, but there is an increasing number that eat in the street again at 3 p.m. and later go back to work for another half shift.

It must be remembered that the Mexican population and that of most of Latin America is undergoing an epidemiological transition that is abruptly leading them from malnutrition to obesity without having ever enjoyed proper nutrition. This is according to their genes and the trend to break with their old lifestyle, which was characterized by healthy physical activity and a diet based on vegetables, whole grains, other seeds, and starchy roots. Mexico's and Latin America's major cities have experienced a huge sudden migration of people, leaving their traditional farming activities and simple diet behind, in exchange for urban food, sometimes they are for their cultural foods, but prepared in different ways [12].

The current situation is possibly even more complex than described above. Probably in the same neighborhood, village or family, children are malnourished, at least moderately, and the parents who were also malnourished are obese, having diabetes, high blood pressure, atherosclerosis or cancer [13]. This is very likely and our research team has shown that people malnourished in childhood become more prone to chronic noncommunicable diseases when adults. It is still unknown to what extent the neglect in street foods is involved in this phenomenon of epidemiological transition.

Social and Economic Issues of Street Food

The activity of selling ready to eat food in stalls or places located in the streets is a large and important economic activity. It is part of the informal economy and has become an employment option for all those who lost their jobs in the recent economic crises. In Mexico City alone, particularly in the last 18 years, sales have expanded across the city, surrounding workplaces, hospitals and clinics, in all sites of heavy traffic, like the downtown area, subway stations, etc. There is practically no broad area, without street food vendors.

The factors most contributing to the increase of street food sales are:

(1) The great rural-urban migration that has filled the periphery of the cities with impoverished populations with a low purchasing power and only occasional employment. The first to arrive are the men, who do not have a place to live and therefore, cooking facilities, so their only option is to buy food in the streets which is easier on their pockets. Since they do not have anywhere to cook and keep what is not used, it is cheaper to eat at street stalls.

(2) The rapid growth of cities force people to commute over long distances from their homes to the workplace and because of their poor purchasing power they cannot afford to go home for meals. This is important in cities like Mexico City with heavy traffic, forcing many people to leave their homes very early, sometimes without any breakfast.

(3) Unemployment has increased substantially, so men and women try to buy and sell and obtain some profit. 'Squatting', living in the street all the time, has already started. The population earning less than twice the minimum wage (about USD 7.00 per family per day) accounts for 56% at the national level and over one third in Mexico City.

(4) The recent recurrent economic crises have led to huge population shifts. The young tend to look for a job in other places. A great change has been seen in food preferences and tastes. In addition to the traditional food in tacos and other variants of corn tortillas, many other foods such as hamburgers and hot dogs are accepted besides packaged cakes, and fried corn, wheat or potato foods.

(5) As a result of the problems of economic adjustments, subsidies for basic commodities are disappearing. For instance, a 400-gram can of sardines used to cost at subsidized prices the equivalent of 20 US cents. This was the favorite food, because of its price and taste, of a large mass of unskilled and occasional workers that worked mainly in the construction industry. A can of sardines was accompanied by tortillas that cost, at subsidized prices of 0.8 US cents per kilo, chili sauces or just chili, sodas or fresh fruit juices of many kinds. Since subsidies are no longer granted, it is cheaper to eat at street stalls that offer a wider variety of food and at times lower prices.

Types of Street Foods Sold

Although most of the street foods are based on tortillas whether as tacos or in an almost infinite variety of forms and presentations, fried, stuffed before frying, big or small, and with different fillings, the fillings in tacos depend on their availability, market price, and local taste. What is sold most is hot tortilla stuffed with some meat, usually fatty pork, beef or various prepared dishes (potatoes alone or with fried chili strips, chicken, ham, headcheese, nopal pads with some type of meat or pork skin, or just sauce, sausages with chili, pork skin with chili, pressed pork skin with chili, blood sausage, or hard-boiled eggs alone or combined with chili, etc.). Most times all these foods are served with rice. The most expensive ones are the most typical ones: mutton ('barbacoa'), fried pork cubes, or steak, or dried cured meat. The most common tacos are 'basket tacos'. They are the most popular because of their price and flavor. They are homemade, and while still hot, are placed in a basket and sold. These are usually tortillas stuffed with beans, pressed pork skin, green 'mole', potatoes, spiced pork, etc. These cooked tacos are carried in wicker baskets covered with a piece of cloth or plastic to keep them warm. For preservation purposes, a large amount of oil is added and apart of their attractiveness is that they are accompanied by red chili sauces made with tomatoes. 'Tamales' are made with the same dough as tortillas, but lard, chili and meat are added. They are cooked in corn husks and are eaten at breakfast out of the home. 'Quesadillas' are slightly thicker tortillas, folded in half and stuffed with vegetables such as mushrooms, squash flowers, corn fungus, or else cheese, pork skin, potatoes with some type of meat or one of the prepared dishes mentioned above.

All street food stalls usually have bowls of chopped onion, cilantro and lime wedges, some even have cucumbers, 'papalo quelite', sliced radish and, of course, all sorts of sauces. Mainly in the coastal towns, there are also fish, octopus, squid and shrimp tacos. Seafood cocktails called 'campechana' are very popular in Mexico, a mixture of shrimp and oysters or a 'life giver', a combination of fish, octopus, squid, marinated fish and different sorts of seafood (shrimp, clams, 'pata de mula', oysters, etc.). Both are served with tomato ketchup, onion, cilantro, chili sauce, avocado and lime juice.

There are other foods in other cities of the country where the sale of street foods has become popular. These are typical local dishes, or in many cases, local specialties of European origin. For example, in Pachuca, the capital of the state of Hidalgo, a city that for a long time was famous for European dishes due to the presence of many British mining engineers. The famous English 'pasties' were adapted and now are very popular under the name of 'pastes', with savory or sweet fillings. Another example of the adaptation of British food to Latin food is 'gingerbread' cookies, which became 'ginyabre' and are very popular in stores and street stalls in some cities of northern Mexico.

In the streets of the city of Oaxaca, toasted grasshoppers (very crunchy) are sold with salt and lemon. Besides being nutritious, they are the delight of Mexicans and foreigners love them. The legs are removed and the body is fried or roasted and eaten in a taco. In Cuernavaca and other cities near Mexico City, 'jumiles' (triatomas) tacos are sold. Curiously enough, these strange little insects are eaten live and escape from the tortilla to walk on the cheeks of the people who enjoy this bizarre delicacy.

Many types of 'tamales' are sold throughout the country. There are many different sorts, types and flavors, made of processed corn dough wrapped in corn husks or banana leaves with chili sauce and a small amount of any type of meat. Sometimes they are eaten in a bread roll and at other times alone, and are accompanied by 'atole', which is a thin corn gruel flavored with different fruits, fruit essences or chocolate. In the latter case it is called 'champurrado'. The combination makes a really tasty, nutritious and cheap breakfast or supper, and so, is favored by certain sectors of the population, though it is eaten by different social classes. Those who can afford to, eat 'tamales' in restaurants and fixed locales. 'Tamale' street stalls may be considered almost as an informal Mexican franchise. They are prepared at home and transported in motor vehicles or carts and are left in previously contracted sites for sale. Very early in the morning the aroma of 'tamales' pervades the city and all classes enjoy them for breakfast.

The product that competes with 'tacos' are 'tortas', a bread roll ('bolillo') halved and filled with cheese, ham, salad vegetables and chili, as well as many other ingredients. They are a complete and usually cheap meal.

Other products are colorful homemade meringues or fruits and vegetables sold from carts in many forms and presentations: pineapple, watermelon, prickly pears, melons, yam beans, cucumbers or mango, some sliced and others, as in the case of the latter two, artistically cut. In particular, mangos are impaled on a small wood stick, while others are cut in pieces and sold in plastic bags. Both slices and pieces are seasoned to taste with salt, powdered chili and lime juice, all being very popular for their flavor. Fruit cocktails, vegetable cocktails, fruit and vegetable juices and flavored waters, decorate the streets with their colors, especially during the summer months.

Some cities, for example, Celaya, display with a wide variety of milk-based candies. Natural vanilla, wine-flavored, or burned caramelized milk, wafers and 'burritas' are some of the most popular ones. They are nutritious, delicious, and inexpensive, and bacteriologically safer because of their high sugar content. In Mexico City, they are sold to drivers who stop at traffic lights.

Fried plantains are always present in coastal towns, as are barbecued shrimp and fish and smelt, eaten fried with or without chili and lime juice.

The large amount and wide variety of crystallized fruits are also worth mentioning: pineapple, coconut, stuffed limes, a wide range of berries and plums, orange skins and lately crystallized vegetables are being sold, such as carrots, beets, nopal pads, eggplants and even chilies. Strange as it may sound, they are delicious.

A long list of strange and exquisite products can be added: 'esquites', fresh corn kernels cooked with epazote (an herb), salt and a little lard to be seasoned with powdered chili and lime juice. Other foods are ears of corn covered with mayonnaise, butter or cream, plus cheese and powdered chili or simply with lime juice, salt and chili; 'sopes', 'flautas', flavored yogurt, 'pambazos', stuffed tamales, pork and hominy stew, chestnuts, sweet fritters, tripe stew and of course, marinated fish cocktails, fried fish, chicken drumsticks, gizzards or liver, flavored shaved ice, cotton candy, etc.

Nutritional Aspects

Much of the food sold on the street contains a large amount of vitamins and minerals and, of course, carotenoids, particularly beta-carotene, lutein and lycopene. Fresh fruits, juices and fresh vegetable cocktails are sold throughout the year and are a rich source of vitamins, beta-carotene, and soluble and insoluble fiber. 'Tacos', 'quesadillas' and 'tortas' are fat-rich foods providing proteins, calories, and also large amounts of other micronutrients such as iron (although not very absorbable), and calcium (because corn tortillas are made with the mineral lime), and various amount of thiamine, riboflavin, niacin and zinc. There is a strong possibility that favorite tropical fruits and vegetables contain bioactive phytochemicals that have not yet been identified or quantified [16].

For higher social classes, street food represents a greater risk, above all, due to pollution and the risk of communicable disease against which they do not have the same level of antibodies. It can also represent a greater risk in the development of chronic diseases, because they add street food containing more fats, particularly the trans type to their regular meals. For low-income groups, street food is not additional food but rather a replacement because it is similar to the food they eat at home, even insofar as pollution is concerned.

Tourists face a special problem, basically in connection with pollution which almost always leads to diarrhea and other severe conditions, the notorious 'Montezuma's revenge', for example. However, it must be made clear that street foods are not always responsible for it. They are indirectly responsible because hotels often buy food from processed products distributors, called 'wholesalers' who pick them up from the homes where they are prepared and thus save money in their own kitchens.

Microbial Quality of Street Foods and Foodborne Diseases

One of the frequent problems of the sale of street foods is their actual and potential hazard caused by bacterial contamination. Unfortunately, there are no adequate data and statistics available. People usually go to the doctor because they have sudden severe diarrhea, but this is not reported to the Ministry of Health. The same happens when they have to go to the hospital because of a severe illness. Both the private physician and health centers such as hospitals must report all cases. However, unless a severe mass food poisoning occurs, nothing is reported. Microbiological contamination comes not only from prepared meals, but also from food kept at room temperature for a long period of time, which turns it into an excellent culture broth. It is quite common that poor quality raw material is used for 'tacos' or 'tortas' or the hands or water used are contaminated. This is very important in many cases, for instance, when fresh fruit juices are prepared. In many cases the primary contamination factors are poorly washed hands of those preparing or serving food. At other times flies can contaminate improperly covered food with feces. Another frequent source of contamination leading to a serious problem is the fact that there are no sanitary facilities available for vendors, such as toilets and washbasins.

In studies conducted at street vendors' stalls sampled by the Ministry of Health, it has been found that food is basically contaminated by coliform organisms clearly indicating a fecal-oral contamination due to the poor hygiene of people handling food or the presence of flies or rodents [17]. The second in importance was staphylococci due to careless handling of food by individuals with rhinopharyngitis or skin lesions. The third problem are fungi and yeasts that point to preservation problems with the resulting deterioration of food. In almost 20% of the samples of meat studied, *Salmonella* or *Shigella* were found. However, the fact that food is cooked before delivering it to the consumer has led to much lower infection rates. In the event of severe mass infections meriting hospitalization and attracting health authorities' attention, it is likely that the most frequent responsible organisms are *Shigella*.

There was a very serious problem in the past that fortunately has been mainly solved: that of additives to give artificial color and flavor to homemade beverages and gelatins. Red dye 2 was used in large quantities but this practice is now under control.

Another persisting problem on its way to being solved is pollution with heavy metals such as lead. Lead comes from the glazed clay pots frequently used in cooking. To a large extent they have already been replaced by steel aluminum pots.

Finally, street dust is another food contamination problem. One of its components is dry feces. Other contaminants are caused by gasoline vapors, diesel and other fuels. Gas and carbon used as fuel to prepare food are also contaminants. For many years, gas was delivered in small tanks which were connected to street carts or movable counters. Pesticide and insecticide pollution are also common, some originating in the fields where the plants are grown, and others in the stalls.

The Health Control Bureau, Ministry of Health, has worked hard in drafting the regulations on the preparation, preservation and handling of street food [18]. There is current regulation in force that employees and managers of street stalls must: (1) have a health card issued after a medical examination has been performed; (2) keep a supply of drinking water sufficient for the day's activities, covered with a lid; (3) the working surface must be waterproof, rustless, and the place must be kept clean including the floor, whether made of wood or the sidewalk, and also the equipment and utensils must be washed with drinking water and soap; (4) waste must be disposed of in covered bins and kept clean; (5) food must be protected from dust, sun and insects; (6) meat, seafood and dairy products must be kept in a refrigerator at a temperature not more than 5 °C. Fresh fruit and vegetables must be washed and disinfected; (7) cooked foods must be kept at 6–7 °C, never at room temperature. They can also be kept in the refrigerator; (8) all food and beverages left by a customer must be disposed of immediately; (9) the staff preparing and serving food must be clean and well-groomed, women must keep their hair short or well tucked up, wear a large white clean coat or apron, and must not handle money. They must wash their hands before preparing and serving food and this as many times as necessary; and, finally (10) all the equipment for food preparation and preservation must be placed at least 2 meters from where pedestrians pass. They should not cause obstruction or nuisance with garbage bins, noise and animals taken to the worksite [19, 20].

These are minimal regulations that are being increasingly observed. However, more training and surveillance are essential. Maybe a simple way is to offer hygiene and food preservation courses and guidance to the public to help people select those businesses that offer greatest safety insofar as quality and cleanliness is concerned. It would be also advisable to provide a telephone number to report offenses and poor food management practices so that the authorities can enforce compliance with regulations.

Profile of Street Vendors and the Role of Women in Street Foods

The sale of food in the streets has become a major business activity and profits can be up to ten times the region's minimum wage. In Mexico City it is estimated that street vendors earn the same as a civil servant working in an office or a professional (fig. 3).

Both men and women work in this activity. Most street vendors are between 20 and 50 years of age with 8 years of formal schooling. However, many illiterate individuals can be found, principally functional illiterates. The signs announcing their products have many misspelled words that are currently quite picturesque, so much so that now we find that many are written wrongly on purpose to attract attention. Their language is very typical of the region where they reside. In Mexico City they have a very special language and accent.

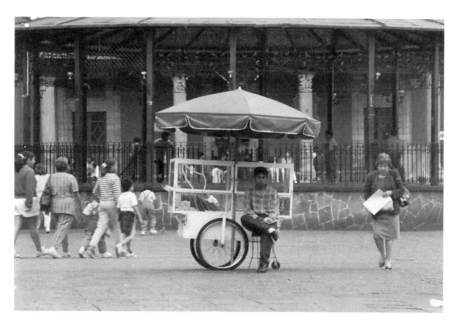

Fig. 3. Typical street vendor at his cart in a square.

It is worth mentioning that their grammatical deficiencies are offset by natural skill: they never make mistakes in charging or giving change, their business accounts are always accurate. They are usually very polite, affable and good tempered. Men and women alike divide task responsibilities. Women cook the food to be sold later in the day, but the men are responsible for buying all that is necessary for the preparation [5, 14].

Women begin work very early in the stalls, because they are the ones who sell 'tamales', cornmeal gruel and 'tacos' at noon. Men usually stay late in the stalls (usually until 10 p.m.). At 'brunch' time they both prepare food and charge. Men are responsible for tidying and cleaning the workplace, constantly washing and cleaning the hotplates where they cook, fry or heat, collecting and disposing of garbage, fetching all the water that is necessary. Women are responsible for washing at home the utensils and dishes used at work. A very important division of labor follows: traditionally, men are the 'taqueros', or the ones that prepare and sell 'tacos', maybe because they feel that 'tacos' are very masculine or maybe because there is a greater demand for 'tacos' at night. In turn, women prepare breakfast dishes, maybe because this is considered more feminine, and so become the main 'tamale' and cornmeal gruel sellers [14].

Processing, Distribution and Wrapping of Street Foods

The food sold at street stalls is prepared at home by those who own or run the stalls. Therefore, it is usually homestyle food. Foods are prepared the night before or in the early hours and the most common containers to transport them are plastic tubs with lids. It is different if food is to be heated later at the point of sale or if it is going to be kept hot without being heated further [5, 14]. At times food is packed in wicker baskets with a first layer of cotton cloth, followed by another plastic (polyethylene) layer and then cotton cloth, and the 'tacos' or 'quesadillas' (turnovers) are placed in layers according to the filling (four or five varieties) and finally they are covered with a sheet of plastic and cotton cloth [15].

'Tamales' are kept in the steamer in which they were cooked, and are usually transported in cars or carts (wheelbarrows and platforms with small wheels) to the point of sale agreed upon. It is worth noting that these are busy points and strangely they are located near hospitals, health centers, etc. The customers are not only patients' relatives, but also the staff of these hospitals and clinics, ranging from physicians to people with minor jobs. The schedule is only for breakfast, between 6 and 9 a.m., but on some sites near markets or even inside the public markets themselves, in some neighborhoods and villages, 'tamales' and cornmeal gruel are served daily between 7 and 11 p.m. for a light supper. Everything is usually sold on the same day, but if there are leftovers, they are fried and sold the next day. Juices are made on site as are flavored waters (fig. 4).

'Tortas' are not transported ready made; they are prepared at the point of sale and only the necessary ingredients are transported. Usually wicker baskets, plastic and paper bags are used and containers at times cooled with ice are used for meat and perishable foods. One of the most popular 'torta' contains breaded veal cutlet, and interestingly the 'tortas' have foreign names according to their ingredients, such as 'Hawaiian' with pineapple, 'German' with sausages, 'Swiss' with cheese, etc. Of course, there are combination and vegetarian 'tortas'. The latter do not contain meat; instead they are made with avocado, cheese, beans and onion. Nothing is sold packaged. Plastic plates with paper napkins or brown paper are provided for 'tortas' to be eaten on site and when they are 'to go' they are well wrapped in paper, napkins or brown paper and put into paper or plastic bags. Cornmeal gruels are served in styrofoam cups with a lid, 'quesadillas' are sold in aluminum foil and styrofoam plates, 'tamales' in their own corn husk envelope, then wrapped in paper and placed in plastic or paper bags. Sodas are usually served in their own bottles, and if beverages are homemade, they are served in plastic or styrofoam cups and a straw may be used or not.

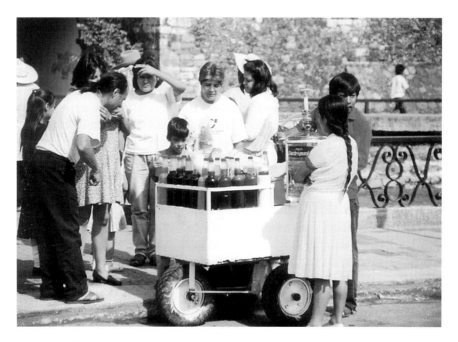

Fig. 4. Fruit juice stand.

Comments, Conclusions and Summary

It is not easy to determine whether street food is more damaging than it is beneficial for health. There is doubt whether there are more negative than positive aspects. From the social and economic points of view this is a great help to workers, who cannot obtain the food they like at affordable prices in regular restaurants. From the health and nutritional points of view, there is no doubt that these meals could and should be presented in better conditions, although if one stops to consider the amount of food necessary and the prices paid, one must admit that it is difficult to offer it in better conditions. It may be concluded that street foods are a necessary evil, important for a city to function. Because of the poverty of the majorities, irregular jobs in time and space, and need for women to find a job, and other socioeconomic factors, it is increasingly difficult to control these foods [3, 4].

There are many factors involved in the proliferation of this unique business: the exodus of a large number of rural inhabitants due to the poor standards of living in their home towns and the resulting unchecked growth of major cities, forcing people to travel long distances between their homes and workplaces. The growing number of students that eat food in the street, the shortage or complete absence of large establishments offering meal facilities for their employees, in addition to the restricted lunch service offered in public schools, the drop in the purchasing power of the population and even nostalgia of those who look for a meal similar to their traditions and customs, as opposed to a hamburger or fried chicken offered by the large international fast-food chains.

There is also the political issue. The sale of street food challenges local and national authorities because sellers invade sidewalks and heaps of garbage disfigure cities. This trade also represents an uncontrolled growth of the underground economy which competes unfairly against regular commerce because vendors do not pay taxes or rent. They also give rise to expenses and overburden the budget which is so necessary to provide public utilities, such as water, electricity and garbage collection. Governments will face a great challenge in the next century: on the one hand, to meet the demand for services, and on the other not to fail to meet public needs [3].

This is already a serious political issue. First to provide food that low-income groups can afford and second, recognize the pressing need of not to ban a basic economic activity for thousands or even millions of people who earn their living by selling raw material, processing foods and selling them in the street.

A reasonable solution would involve limiting sales areas, with better sanitation, with health and nutritional education for vendors and consumers and constant surveillance and supervision of product quality. In recent years, the situation has been very dynamic in Mexico City and in many other capital cities of Latin America. Health and nutritional improvements are evident, perhaps due to the competition among the vendors themselves and in some countries as a result of government action. However, the increase of sales in streets has been huge and chaotic to a large extent. Consumers are unable to control this because at this time they do not realize that they are creating a serious problem that only they can solve. Therefore, the tool that governments have to regulate this very special and problematic market is consumer education, nutritional education in all aspects and places – schools, media, women's organizations, etc. This way not only several problems arising from the sale of street foods could be solved, but others, such as nutrition of the public in general and that of the most vulnerable groups, the risk of child malnutrition and chronic diseases of the elderly.

References

1   Chauliac M: Implications of Street Foods for Children. Rome, FAO, 1995.
2   Rocabado QF, Bermejo MS: Diagnóstico sobre la situación de la protección de los alimentos en México. Secretaría de Salud, OPS/OMS. Mexico, 1993.
3   Alba F: La población de México: Evolución y dilemas. México, El Colegio de México, 1987, p 189.
4   Avila A, Shamah T, Chávez A: Encuesta urbana de alimentación y nutricion en la zona metropolitana de la Cd. de México, ENURBAL 1995. México, Publ División de Nutrición, 1996.
5   FAO: Food and nutrition investigation, No 63. Rome, 1995.
6   Alman L: Historia de México, 5 vol. México, Ed JUS col. Grandes autores mexicanos, 1942.
7   Espinosa CLM: Contribución al estudio del hambre en la sociedad novohispana durante el siglo XVIII. México, Ed CONACYT-INN, 1986.
8   Gonzalez Casanova P (coord): Historia del hambre en México. México, Ed Instituto Nacional de la Nutrición, 1987.
9   Lisker R, Perez BJ, Granados B, Babinsky J, De Rubens S, Armendares S, Buentello B: Gene frequencies and admixture estimates in Mexico City population. Am J Phys Anthropol 1986;71: 203.
10 Chávez A, Muñoz Ch M, Roldan JA, Bermejo S, Avila A: La nutrición en México y la transición epidemiológica. Foro alimentación y nutrición. México, Instituto Nacional de la Nutrición, 1993.
11 Secretariá de Salud: La incidencia de las enfermedades trasmitidas por alimentos, Capítulo X de diagnóstico sobre la situación de la protección de los alimentos en México; in Rocabado QF, Bermejo MS (eds): Secretaría de Salud. México, OPS/OMS, 1993.
12 Chávez A, Muñoz Ch M, Roldán JA, Bermejo S, Avila A, Madrigal H: The food and nutrition situation of Mexico: A food consumption, nutritional status and applied programs tendencies, report from 1960 to 1990. Subdireccion de Nutricion, Instituto Nacional de la Nutricion. Mexico, Ed PAX, 1996.
13 Chávez A, Muñoz Ch M: La nueva alimentación, libro ed. México, PAX 1995.
14 Secretaría de Salud, Dirección General de Control Sanitario, La venta de alimentos en la vía pública, México, 1992.
15 Romero Torres J: Appropriate Technologies Appllied to Street Foods. Rome, FAO, 1995.
16 Muñoz de Ch M, Chávez A, Roldán JA, Ledesma JA Pérez-Gil F, Mendoza E: Valor nutritivo de los alimentos de mayor consumo en México, Editorial. México, PAX, 1996.
17 Beltrán PF: Análisis de factores de riesgo y determinación de puntos críticos de control en el procesamiento de alimentos. Colombia, Publ Universidad de Antioquía, 1988.
18 Servicios de salud Pública del distrito federal: Manual de procedimientos de regulación sanitaria. México, SSA, 1989.
19 Dirección de Regulación Sanitaria: Requisitos sanitarios para expendios ambulantes y semifijos de alimentos. México, Ed Secretaría de Salud, Dirección de Regulación y Fomento Sanitario, 1991.
20 Diario Oficial de la Federación: Organo del Gobierno Constitucional de los Estados Unidos Mexicanos, México, D.F. Lunes 18 de Enero, 1988.

Miriam Muñoz de Chávez, National Cancer Institute, National Nutrition Institute,
National School of Anthropology and History, Metropolitan University, Xochimilco (Mexico)

Simopoulos AP, Bhat RV (eds): Street Foods.
World Rev Nutr Diet. Basel, Karger, 2000, vol 86, pp 155–168

....

Street Food Vending: The Israeli Scenario

Liora Gvion-Rosenberg[a], *Naomi Trostler*[b]

[a] Department of Behavioral Sciences, Kibbutzim, Tel-Aviv, and
[b] School of Nutritional Sciences, Institute of Biochemistry, Food Science and Nutrition, Faculty of Agricultural, Food and Environmental Quality Sciences, Hebrew University of Jerusalem, Rehovot, Israel

In its earliest years after its establishment in 1948, the state of Israel had some of the preconditions for the development of street foods: a high industrialization rate along with long working hours, recruitment of women and men into the labor market, massive immigration in search of employment, and a tendency to spend a lot of time at outdoor activities. Yet, these conditions did not encourage the development of street foods. Moreover, the definition of street foods in Israel differs from that of the 1989 Food and Agriculture Organization (FAO) which states that 'Street foods are ready-to-eat foods and beverages prepared and/or sold by vendors and hawkers especially in streets and other similar public places' [1]. We claim that the street food scene in Israel differs in three aspects: (1) the absence of street vendors in the busy sections of the major cities in favor of small and institutionalized businesses; (2) the lack of an ethnic foods culture or a significant ethnic-oriented economy, and (3) the limited role of women as food vendors.

Wandering around the streets of the major cities in Israel, one will not encounter individual vendors or street carts, but rather small businesses which offer either hot or cold ready-to-go dishes and/or dishes for in-place consumption. These establishments lack the ambience of dining, fancy decorum or high quality food [2]. Food is judged by the degree to which it satisfies hunger and by the efficiency of service. Some of the businesses develop into food chains; other businesses limit their offerings to contemporary culinary fashions which once unfashionable, are either changed to a new repertoire or they close the business.

Unlike other countries, whose culinary offerings have been enriched by the foods of the many immigrants and ethnic groups living in the country [3], the process of integrating ethnic food into the public culinary sphere in Israel has been slow and selective. Due to strong enforcement of the Zionist ideology, which has urged many immigrants to assimilate by obliterating their cultural heritage and culinary traditions [4], food vendors often offered that which was widely perceived as 'Israeli food'.

The traditional roles of women in the household on the one hand and their recruitment to the labor market limited their need to apply their domestic cooking skills as part of an ethnic-based economy [5] in order to make a living. This further explains the absence of women from the public culinary scene.

These factors, we argue, make street foods in Israel a unique case. Our objective is twofold. We will discuss the reasons behind the nonacceptance of street foods as generally defined, and we will describe the 'Israeli street food'.

Economic, religious, social and ethnic practices influence the definition of street food in Israel. Although Israel is part of the industrial world which involves long hours and daily commuting, street vendors have never played an active role in food provision for several reasons. First, climatic conditions (mainly during the summer) generally promote closure of service-oriented work places for 3 h at midday, thus enabling those employees living in the vicinity of their work to return home for the midday meal. Secondly, the majority of work places provide subsidized meals and snacks for their employees. Thirdly, many still bring a homemade, prepackaged meal, often including a hot drink. As such, street cart vending is unprofitable and street food is generally limited to snacks and extras which are not regarded as meals. Consequently, the context of street food in Israel is different.

The role of women in the Middle East social realm has prevented them from contributing to the household income because of a traditional notion delineating the social boundaries between the domestic and the public spheres. Consequently, Israel lacks an ethnic-based street food economy, traditionally carried out by women who used their domestic skills for the preparation and selling of ethnic dishes in order to contribute to the household earnings. Women were to be domestically active, leaving the role of 'bread winning' to their husbands. Moreover, cooking and serving food in public was by-and-large regarded as unacceptable and contradictory to the established role for women. These norms coincided with the religious perspective that has limited the role and status of women to home and family [6].

Although Israeli culture is enriched by immigrants from a variety of ethnic backgrounds, including those coming from an environment of street food economy, the concept of street food in their traditional format has not been transplanted into the local food scene. The culture and foods of non-European newcomers were overshadowed by their European counterparts; what has emerged is now crystallizing into the 'Israeli culinary culture'. This course was unlike the process in other parts of the world where immigrants have exercised their culinary knowledge as a potential source of income, especially for women [5, 7]. Moreover, unlike immigrants in most developed countries where recent changes have bolstered newly found pride in national and ethnic foods that once lacked social prestige [8], ethnic foods in Israel have never been part of the country's culinary culture until recently, because of the national dream to create a homogeneous state and culture.

The History of Street Foods

Culturally, meals are an integral part of family life. Research indicates that meals have a major role in the construction or destruction of family life. Recent divorcees and newly remarried individuals report that meals in their previous marriage were more of a battle scene than a pleasant family gathering, whereas in their new relationship meals are a central event of the day and an opportunity to share the daily events with the rest of the family [9]. Ellis [10] showed that battered wives were often beaten up when failing to prepare and serve a hot meal upon the husband's return home. Murcott [11–13] reported about the laborious preparations taken by either fully employed women or housewives to prepare a 'meat, potato, and vegetable' hot dinner in order to please their husbands. None of the women bothered to ask themselves why they did so. They all assumed it was part of their domestic duties.

Meals have always been an important element in Israeli tradition and family life; they either have been eaten at home or at the work place where a close approximation to traditional home cooking has been made. Meals are a major element of the Jewish tradition as well. They are the center of major holidays, rites of passage and major life events. Bound by strict dietary laws they are thoroughly structured in order to prevent the mixture of milk and meat-type dishes and utensils. At the same time, to answer the globalization of eating style, novel culinary products are introduced, i.e. dairy-free 'milk' and 'cream' enable the preparation of milk- and cream-based sauces and desserts into the menu. 'Eating out' has been reserved for either special occasions calling for festive dishes or for consumption of a cuisine not part of the customary diet. As the time required for commuting and the work hours with shorter breaks has increased, an appreciable segment of the population has eliminated breakfast along with the traditional midday main meal consumed at home. This resulted in the establishment of a host of cafeterias, kiosks, or restaurants which have provided alternatives in and around the work place rather than street foods. Traditional meal patterns have not been broken nor replaced by commercial snacks, as has happened in other industrialized countries [2].

Paradoxically, developments in technology and the growing industrialization of the culinary sphere contributed to the domination of the midday main meal rather than to its substitution by street foods. Many households have chosen to incorporate ready-made convenience foods, easily prepared or heated in the microwave oven, into the home-cooked meals. Children can prepare their own hot meals at home, thus reducing their reliance on fast foods and street foods.

Even in the early years of the state of Israel, in the 1950s and 1960s, during which Israelis experienced economic hardship, street foods were never integrated into the daily meal pattern. Street vendors offered, mostly on the beach promenade, town squares or street corners, a very small repertoire of snack foods, such as *falafel* (chick pea balls, ground and fried), corn on the cob (boiled, served in its husk with plenty of salt), sunflower seeds (dried and salted), ice cream, or *gazoz* (soda water with fruit flavors). These were regarded as 'between meal' snacks because the Israeli Central and Eastern European middle class, in whose culture it was utterly impolite to eat in the street, rejected the 'falafel culture' and what it represented.

The 1970s brought about changes in the national economy, standard of living and culture, and even to the selection of snack foods. More Israelis traveled abroad and their exposure to a variety of foreign foods affected demand for foods not regularly consumed at home. *Malaby* (a sweet pudding with almond flavor), corn, and ice cream cones disappeared in favor of pizza and *shawarma* (meat broiled on a spit and eaten in pita bread) counters. Furthermore, hamburgers, steak sandwiches, and fast food establishments became popular rather than street foods consumed on the street.

The new foods served similar functions. First, while the economic shortages in the early years of the state of Israel dictated a daily diet low in meat consumption, the new dishes symbolized the changes in the national economy which included a growing consumption of meat. Secondly, the foods were associated with the diet, eating habits, and the standard of living of the middle class, and food items of the lower classes were disregarded. Thirdly, the changes in the culinary scene coincided with a cultural trend largely referred to as 'the Americanization' of Israeli society. An attempt to imitate all that was associated with the American culture had its gastronomic manifestations. Hamburgers on a bun served with french fries, ketchup, and Coca-

Cola signified for many the domination of the American culture over the Mediterranean culture.

During the 1980s another change took place distancing the Israeli public gastronomic sphere even more from the typical street vendor. An additional rise in the standard of living and a growing number of households which enjoyed a relatively high dual income encouraged the consumption of ready-made meals, exotic dishes, and ethnic foods. This was the age of fast food chains and 'boutiques' for breads, bagels (American influence), baguettes and croissants (French influence), *Ziva* (baked dough rings stuffed with cheese or mushrooms) and *jachnun* (dough rolled over itself, baked overnight – both latter items are a Yemenite influence), *bureka* (phyllo dough stuffed with either feta cheese, hard cheese, potatoes, mushrooms or spinach – a Middle East influence), and a variety of pita breads (associated with the emerging ethnic revival of the immigrants from the Middle East region), which were opened by young, world-traveled, entrepreneurs. It is important to note that although these foods were quite popular because of their nature and price, and the recognition of ethnic groups for their contribution to the culinary scene was increasing, the foods catered mostly to the middle class.

The rise in the standard of living, the growing percentage of working mothers, and recent technological developments such as the microwave oven reduced the amount of daily cooking in the home. Domestic cooking became part of leisure and was limited to the weekends. Yet the midday meal was still perceived as the main meal of the day. The ability to allow children to choose their own lunch at a fast food place became a common feature of the middle class lifestyle. The lower class could also periodically afford to eat out and purchase ready-made foods. Their attempts to imitate the lifestyle of the middle class contributed to making the purchase of ready-made foods socially acceptable to replace the homemade meal.

The 1990s introduced what one may call the 'Yuppie era', young professionals, mainly third generation of immigrants who no longer feared to admit a longing for their traditional ethnic dishes. They were the economically well off, upwardly mobile group of society. This era has consisted of two supplementing trends. Exotic foods such as *sushi, sashimi,* muffins, seven-grain breads, tofu, and sophisticated ice creams, now dominate the public culinary scene and have become an integral part of the repertoire. These foods are all purchased from counters associated with well-established restaurants. At the same time, ethnic Arab dishes are attracting their share of the public, mainly on the grounds of their good health promotion qualities. *Humus* (a chick pea paste), *tahini* (a sesame seed paste), and *falafel* have made a comeback.

The Socioeconomic Aspects of Street Foods

As noted, street food vendors, as seen in developing countries, are not part of the Israeli gastronomic scene. Ready-to-eat foods are manufactured and processed by food industries, home industries, caterers or restaurateurs. The Israeli street foods share the following characteristics:

(1) They are sold as fast foods and dry snack food. Chocolate bars, cheese or peanut 'doodles', potato chips, or nuts are all regarded as food to be purchased from kiosks or from vending machines.

(2) They are considered snacks, not an integral part of the meal pattern. A sandwich consumed during lunchtime, for example, is not perceived as a meal in itself even if it contains all the major elements of a meal such as cold cuts, cheese, eggs or fish (protein and fat); bread (carbohydrates); and fresh vegetables (fiber and micronutrients). As one is expected to dine properly on a 'meat, potato, and vegetable' meal, a sandwich is defined as a snack to be consumed at all times.

(3) The variety of foods reflects the changes in the economic and cultural aspects of life in Israel. The higher the standard of living, the greater the variety and sophistication of foods, as seen in the previous section. Moreover, the repertoire reflects upon changes in the taste and eating style of the middle class.

(4) Changes in the repertoire coincide with technological developments, i.e. the freezer and the microwave oven which have made it possible to serve precooked meals.

(5) The introduction of pizza, *sushi*, or sophisticated ice creams, to mention only a few, was preceded by exposure to foreign foods and cultures during the travels of Israelis abroad, and are an expression of the tendency to imitate and assimilate these experiences and favorite new foods. In Israel, the well-to-do are the first to integrate foreign influences into their eating and entertainment habits. Later on this pattern is imitated (and adapted) by the lower economic classes.

(6) Foods sold on the street reflect the current consumer trends and thus cater to middle class taste. Whereas the lower class may lack the economic means to consume rather expensive snacks, the middle class searches for sophisticated and exotic foods. For example, this search has resulted in the introduction of stores which sell a variety of fancy breads, some of which are quite expensive, *sushi* bars, and sandwich bars where a customer creates his or her own sandwich from many choices, from the conventional to the exotic, starting with the bread through the spread, selecting major and minor items, and ending with different kinds of vegetable toppings. The lower class would more likely look for *humus* served in whole wheat or fiber-enriched

pita bread, plain egg or cheese sandwiches, or pizza with unconventional toppings.

(7) Regardless of the types of food sold, they are all made available through commercial outlets, except for a few vendors of seasonal foods such as corn on the cob or ice cream bars.

Types of Street Foods Sold on Regular and Special Occasions

The Israeli version of street foods is generally available at kiosks and shops. *Falafel*, sunflower seeds, nuts, ice cream, or pizza, are all part of the daily culinary street scene. Until recently, the quest for assimilation and negation of other ethnic cultures resulted in the lack of authentic ethnic street foods. As of the 1980s, the growing social legitimacy for immigrants to express and develop their individual ethnic identity, allowed for the gradual introduction and acceptance of ethnic foods. The following are but a few of the now well received ethnic foods which enrich the repertoire of street foods in Israel: *sambusak* (vegetable or meat pie; a dish of Iraqi origin), *couscous* (a rice-like dish made of semolina; of North African origin), *Druze pita* (a very thin flat bread), 'Arab delights' such as *baklava* (phyllo dough filled with nuts and honey), and a wide assortment of Russian breads.

In parallel, new trends have emerged, specifically, events known as 'Food Fairs'. Thematic and nonthematic food fairs are currently capturing the attention of the public. Their popularity indicates the interest of the public to expand its 'culinary horizons' by exposure to new foods and to learn how to incorporate specialty foods into their regular menus.

Nonthematic food fairs are generally weekly events. Local, small domestic industries supply most of the foodstuffs. Wandering among the stands, one can taste and purchase ethnic dishes, as well as their adaptations to mainstream tastes, novel foods like *sushi*, and a variety of cottage industry products, such as breads, jams and marmalades, fruits and fruit juices, fresh garden vegetables, stuffed vegetables, hot soups, salads, sandwiches, and vegetable-based novelty ice creams.

Take, for example, a nonthematic food fair which takes place every Friday noon at a central shopping mall. Visitors stop for breakfast or lunch in one of the small food places. The food fair seems to fulfill the interest and curiosity of mall visitors. For one, it enables customers to taste and shop for unconventional products and become acquainted with homemade dishes. Secondly, it exposes the customers to personal encounters with small manufacturers. It also is an opportunity to familiarize oneself with a variety of dishes other than those offered at the major food chains. Thirdly, it enables food fair producers to establish a clientele which frequents the mall on a regular basis. Some of the customers set their orders a week in advance or on the telephone and arrive to pick up merchandise.

The variety of food items, dishes and producers further indicates the unique case of street food in Israel. In addition to vendors and entrepreneurs, restaurateurs, who already have licensed local industries, take the opportunity to offer samples of their specialties at food fairs. Let us discuss a few examples: two entrepreneurs who participate at the food fair at the Dizengoff Center Shopping Mall (located in the center of Tel-Aviv) own small and simple restaurants in the mall itself, namely the 'Boston Deli' and 'Druze Food' (Druz are an Arab sect). Both are self-service places which offer full meals as either American or Middle East type dishes at relatively low prices. At the food fair stands they offer relatively inexpensive small samples. Despite the fact that the two are well established, they use the fair as a potential attraction for their style of food and main location. Other well-established entrepreneurs are the owner of a popular bakery located across the street from the mall, and a well-known vegetarian Indian restaurant located in a smaller shopping mall close by. Although the two are well-known establishments in the local culinary scene and have established a reputation as well as devoted clientele, they feel that curious customers can always be attracted. The bakery offers fresh-baked novel breads, while the Indian restaurant limits its variety to appetizers such as vegetable *samosa* (fried wheat pastry turnover stuffed with potato and peas) or *pakora* (vegetables dipped in batter and deep fried).

Thematic food fairs are 'culinary based' and generally are annual fairs held in central city venues or parks. Cheese, bread, wine, ice cream, and chocolate fairs are recent examples. These events are sponsored by either food industries or private businesses. Stalls are run by professional chefs and restaurateurs, as well as nonprofessional food vendors, young entrepreneurs, and food industry representatives. All seek to attract new clientele by offering snacks and samples of sophisticated foods at reasonable prices. The attendees are exposed to foods and dishes not regularly available.

The Profile of the Israeli Street Vendor

Street food vendors in developing countries are mostly working class women who make their living by expanding their domestic kitchen. Street food vendors in Israel are mostly middle class, yet, their heterogeneous backgrounds reflect upon diversified cultural and culinary traits, various attitudes toward street foods and a distinct commitment to food marketing.

We recognize several groups of street food vendors in the Israeli population. In the 1950s the majority of the street food vendors were immigrants of lower class background. Men would stand on a street corner offering corn on the cob or wander through the streets selling *malaby*. Food vending was either a major or a supplementary source of income. In either case, it was regarded as a temporary means to make a living. Once the vendor accumulated enough capital, street vending was abandoned in favor of opening an established food place. Such was the case of a popular *bureka* vendor. Upon immigration, the founder of the present chain resided in a two-room apartment. One of the rooms served as living quarters for the family, while in the other he established the bakery. Riding his bicycle, he sold hot *bureka*. When times improved economically for him, he opened a little shop, one shop followed another, and soon enough he became the owner of a major food chain.

A second group consists of restaurateurs who, in addition to their high-priced restaurants have also opened kiosks offering several of the items served at the restaurants at a lower price and simpler ambience. A Japanese-style restaurant opened a simple *sushi* bar next door, and a French-style restaurant opened a French creperie.

A third group of vendors sell food on a part-time basis from door to door. They include students who bake and prepare sandwiches, homemakers known for their culinary skills who have decided to publicly market their wares, and women who cook according to customers' requests. This group has emerged in the past 15 years as a response to the dual career lifestyle which has dominated middle class families. Although working full time, many have not abandoned the daily family meal. Moreover, entertaining peers has remained a major form of leisure activity, one which involves serving of food. Consequently, many professionals choose to order ready-made foods with a homemade flavor. These part-time vendors have established a clientele, mostly by word of mouth, due to their specialties. Unlike the vendors who eventually open their own place leaving the actual cooking in favor of managing a business, the latter wished to quit their regular jobs in favor of making their living from cooking.

Such is the case of a former English teacher, known among her friends for her baked goods. What started as a favor to a friend who asked her to bake a cake for a son's birthday, shortly developed into a business. One order followed another and she was baking three afternoons a week for regular customers. Though she continued working part time, a year later she quit as she was baking full time for four cafes.

The fourth group mainly consists of young women who prepare basic snacks, such as sandwiches, small salads, or cakes, and offer them regularly in work establishments. They engage in food vending as part-time activities to supplement their income. Some of the women establish a stable relationship with organized work places, guaranteeing exclusiveness. Others sell to an occasional customer. This service may replace the breakfast no longer consumed at home or provide occasional snacks.

The Role of Women in Street Foods

Unlike developing countries where women dominate the preparation and the selling of street foods [1, 14], women in Israel, influenced by economic, social and religious customs, have generally refrained from participating in the professional gastronomic scene.

Structurally and culturally speaking, men have always been regarded as the breadwinners, an assumption that excluded women from the business world and set them either in the domestic sphere as semiprofessional cooks in family-owned enterprises. Even then, their cooking was limited to traditional-style dishes rather than creative cooking [15–17]. Thus, when women began to compete professionally in food preparation, they either worked as cooks in cafeterias or established their own small business, rather than becoming street food vendors. This not only guaranteed income, but coincided with the cultural traits, position, and prestige of Israeli women.

A recent change is taking place. Women occupy a greater part in the public culinary scene, mostly through the last two groups of entrepreneurs mentioned in the previous section. Women were the first to offer their home-made goods for sale. Encouraged by their success, they started expanding their clientele and became major suppliers of cafes and restaurants, earning a better income than what they used to earn in their previous jobs.

It is important to note that the first group consists of women in their 40s and 50s who bring their domestic experience into the culinary sphere. These women have chosen to trade their career in favor of a traditional occupation in a new guise. The second group is different. For one, the women are younger, most of them being in their mid- and late 20s. Secondly, they define their occupation as temporary and have no intention of pursuing a career in the catering business. Thirdly, they do not define themselves as chefs or cooks and have no special training, but rather respond to a certain need in the food market. They are not known for their creative cooking but for their simple homemade cooking.

Nutritional Quality of Street Foods

The nature of the Israeli trend in street foods, as described in the previous sections, includes two major characteristics. Firstly, it is an established and organized activity, mainly localized in commercial urban centers. Secondly, it is mainly for snacking purposes, and does not conform to the FAO definition because it is neither prepared nor sold by street vendors and hawkers. Being snack food by definition, street food in Israel does not make an important contribution to essential nutrient intake except to energy from complex and simple carbohydrates and fat. *Falafel, shawarma*, and fruit juices are exceptions. The former provide some protein, and the latter provide select micronutrients. Although some of the food items could provide nutritionally complete meals, they are rarely defined as such. The socially accepted definition of the home-cooked meal (even if purchased) still overrides the nutritional definition.

The more common and popular street foods are prepared by the commercial food industry. Therefore, the nutritional composition will not appreciably vary or differ within the product group. Specialty items prepared by individual connoisseurs would be expected to vary in composition, but they have little impact on the overall nutrient intake, except for energy, as the quantities consumed are relatively small.

To date, no study has been performed from which one could learn about the eating habits and customs of street foods in Israel. The nutritional composition of the food groups regarded as street foods in Israel is: (I) Foods which contribute mainly energy: (a) Baked items – rolls, bagels, plain and sweet rolls, cupcakes, etc., and (b) Sweets and chocolates. (II) Mixed nutrient foods which contribute mainly energy and some protein: (a) Sandwiches, including *falafel*, hard cheeses, cold meats, sardines, *humus*, etc.; (b) hamburgers; (c) pizza; (d) dry snacks, i.e. popcorn, potato chips, nuts, sunflower seeds; (3) ice cream. None of the above food items could be considered as a provider of an appreciable amount of any vitamin, mineral, or microelement, when consumed infrequently in reasonable amounts.

Fresh fruit juices have gained popularity over the years. Fresh fruit juices such as citrus and carrot are available year round, while strawberry and mango, for example, are available fresh only for a short season. Still, these juices would supply energy as well as ample amounts of vitamin C, beta-carotene, potassium and calcium.

Several recent trends in street food consumption may have future impact on overall nutrient intake and should be watched. First, instant minimeals and soups are entering the market and gaining popularity. By law, the nutrient composition of these items has to be on the label. Since they are advertised as replacing a home-cooked meal, their nutrient content is expected to be proportionally adequate. Second, a growing number of large institutions have recently started to introduce minicafeterias, or complimentary well-stocked kitchenettes in central locations on the premises so that the employees arriving early or leaving late will have light snacks to replace the omitted breakfast and nourishment in the late afternoon hours. Here, the variety is diverse and, in part, depends on the negotiation between the employees and the management, or on the latter solely. Since the items consumed could account for meals, their nutritional contribution, in the long run, could impact total nutrient composition. Third, freelance vendors of sandwiches, cupcakes and sweet rolls are frequenting work places. These items might change from a nonhabitual snack to replace a balanced breakfast or any other meal, thereby potentially jeopardizing the overall nutritional intake.

Microbial Contamination

There is no record of there ever being an outbreak of disease that could be traced back to consumption of contaminated street food in Israel. The most prevalent street foods are baked products with a low moisture content due to high heat treatment which support bacterial growth less readily than high moisture foods. Also, the locals are licensed, and food preparation and handling practices are regulated and controlled by municipal authorities. They are required to maintain hygienic practices so as not to pose short-term (bacterial epidemic) as well as long-term (degraded fatty acids in deep-fat frying) public health threats.

Chemical Contamination

The food industry is very tightly regulated. Strictly observed limits exist regarding chemical additives, such as colorants and preservatives, and contaminants such as pesticide residues.

Regulatory Aspects

All food-related activity is licensed and regulated by the local municipality. Street vending of any kind, including food, is regulated through personal licensing. Shops of all types including stands, stalls and kiosks are required to obtain a license. The code for hygienic practices is quite detailed and supervisors perform spot checks unannounced.

Conclusion

In developing countries, street food vending seems to be on the rise. The reasons for this trend are a growing marginal urban population, unemployment, lengthening commutes for workers, a demand for low-cost and culturally appropriate food near the work place and a dire shortage of regular establishments serving such foods. In Israel, street food vending did not gain momentum and has not become an integral contributor to the daily food intake. It is the reason why the role of street foods in supplying nutrients has received little attention.

Unlike developing countries where street foods provide an affordable source of food throughout the day, and are consumed regularly and consistently in place of meals [1], in Israel they are mostly snacks which are relatively expensive and certainly not purchased by the low-income group. They are ready-to-eat in some cases, prepared by formal food industries, or prepared from scratch (sandwiches), or need only the final touch on the spot while waiting at the vendor. There is no 'on the street' food preparation.

Food 'to go' has become most popular in Israel and might replace a home-cooked meal, but it is not consumed on the street and certainly is not consumed by the low-income group. Street food in Israel has developed different characteristics over time, lending itself to specialties ethnic dishes. Changes in the labor market and the economic structure along with exposure to ethnic cultures and world culinary trends has resulted in a growing culinary repertoire, part of which could be defined as street food. Due to the processes mentioned earlier, some foods previously considered 'home cooked' or 'restaurant' food have redefined their status as street foods.

References

1   Draper A: Street Foods in Developing Countries: The Potential for Micronutrient Fortification. US Agency for International Development (USAID), Contract HRN-5122-C-00-3025-00, 1996.
2   Finkelstein J: Dining Out. New York, New York University Press, 1989.
3   Taylor DS, Fishell VK, Derstine JL, Morgan RL, Patterson NR, Moriarty KW, Battista BA, Ratcliffe HE, Binkoski AE, Kris-Etherton PM: Street foods in America: A true melting pot. World Rev Nutr Diet. Basel, Karger, 2000, vol 86, pp 25–44.
4   Swirski S: Education in Israel: Schooling for Inequality (in Hebrew). Tel Aviv, Breirot, 1990.
5   Dallalfar A: Iranian women as immigrant entrepreneurs. Gender Soc 1994;8:541–561.
6   Zubaida S, Tapper R: Culinary Cultures of the Middle East. London, Tauris, 1996.
7   Massey D: The settlement process among Mexican migrants to the United States. Am Soc Rev 1986;51:771–784.
8   Chase H: The Meyhane or McDonald's? Changes in eating habits and the evolution of fast food in Istanbul; in Zubaida S, Tapper R (eds): Culinary Cultures in the Middle East. London, Tauris, 1996, pp 73–86.

9 Burgoyne J: Food and family reconstruction; in Murcott A (ed): Sociology of Food and Eating. Cardiff, Gower, 1983, pp 152–163.

10 Ellis R: The way to a man's heart: Food in the violent home; in Murcott A (ed): Sociology of Food and Eating. Cardiff, Gower, 1983, pp 164–171.

11 Murcott A: Cooking and the cooked: A note on the domestic preparation of meals; in Murcott A (ed): Sociology of Food and Eating. Cardiff, Gover, 1983, pp 178–185.

12 Murcott A: It's a pleasure to cook for him; in Garmaniko D (ed): The Public and the Private. London, Heinman Educational Books, 1983, pp 78–90.

13 Murcott A: On the social significance of the cooked dinner in South Wales. Soc Sci Inform 1982; 21:677–693.

14 Fischler C: Food Habits, social change and the nature/culture dilemma. Soc Sci Inform 1980;19: 937–953.

15 Banner L: Why women have not been great chefs. S Atlantic Q 1973;72:198–212.

16 Frosterman L: Food and celebrations: A kosher caterer as mediator of communal traditions; in Keller Brown L (ed): Ethnic and Regional Foodways in the United States. Knoxville, University of Tennessee Press, 1984, pp 127–142.

17 Gvion L: The Political Aspects of the Arab Cuisine in Israel. Beit Bert, The Institute for Israeli Arab Studies, in press.

Liora Gvion-Rosenberg, Department of Behavioral Sciences,
The Academic College of Tel-Aviv-Yaffo, 4 Antokolosky Street, IL–64044 Tel-Aviv (Israel)
Tel. +972 8 948 1265, Fax +972 8 947 6189

Author Index

Subject Index

Consumers, street foods (continued)
  Australia 51
  Latin America
    education about food safety 135, 136
    food selection factors 127
    income percentage devoted to street
      foods 125
    occupations 126
  United States 41
Corn-on-the-cob, Greek street food
  marketing 11, 12, 18

Doner, Greek street food marketing 8

Fuel sources, street vendors
  Africa 111   Asia 68, 69
  Latin America 127

Greece, street foods
  chemical and microbiological quality
    cheese pies 19, 21
    data sources 19
    gyros 20, 21
    improvement 20
    nuts, seeds, and raisins 21, 22
    souvlaki 19–21
  cities
    Athens 5, 6, 13
    Constantinople 4, 5
    Smyrna 5
    Thessaloniki 13
  consumption and socioeconomics 13–15
  definition of street foods 2
  demand 1
  history 1–6
  nutritional value
    gyros 17, 18
    koulouri 16
    pies 16, 17
    souvlaki 17, 18
  processing, distribution, and packaging
    15, 16
  types
    boyatsa 4
    candy floss 5, 11
    cheese pies 3, 4, 10, 16
    corn-on-the-cob 11, 12, 18

doner 8
gyros 7, 10, 14, 22
koulouri 3, 10, 12, 14, 16
nuts, seeds, and raisins 11, 18
souvlaki 7, 10, 14, 22
vendors
  economics 15
  gender 13
  licensing 13
  numbers 12
  regulation 18, 19
  site selection 11, 12
Gyros
  chemical and microbiological quality
    20, 21
  Greek street food marketing 7, 10, 14, 22
  nutritional value 17, 18

Hazard Analysis and Critical Control Point
  American street foods 37, 38
  Asian street foods 88–90
  background 37

Israel, street foods
  chemical quality 166
  comparison with other countries
    155–157, 167
  definition of street foods 155, 156, 167
  history 157–159
  microbial quality 166
  nutritional quality 164–166
  regulation 166
  socioeconomic aspects 160, 161
  types and venues 161, 162
  vendor profile 162–164
  women, roles 155, 156, 164

Koulouri
  Greek street food marketing
    3, 10, 12, 14, 16
  nutritional value 16

Latin America, street foods, *see also* Mexico,
  street foods
  chemical quality 131
  consumers
    education about food safety 135, 136

location selection 130
raw materials 127
regulation 134, 135
training 135, 136
vehicles 130, 131
waste disposal 130
water sources 129, 130
Mexico City
education levels 149, 150
income 149

regulation 148, 149, 153
sex roles 150
United States
ethnicity 26, 40
gender 40, 41
Internal Revenue Service targeting
39, 40
operating hours 41
regulation 25–27, 38–40
restaurant formation 27, 28